A HOSPICE
GUIDE BOOK

A HOSPICE GUIDE BOOK

HOSPICE CARE:
A Wise Choice Providing Quality Comfort Care
Through the End of Life's Journey

Dr. Curtis E. Smith, Ph.D., Psy.D.

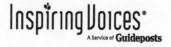
Inspiring Voices®
A Service of Guideposts

Inspiring Voices books may be ordered through booksellers or by contacting:

Inspiring Voices
1663 Liberty Drive
Bloomington, IN 47403
www.inspiringvoices.com
1-(866) 697-5313

ISBN: 978-1-4624-0013-3 (e)
ISBN: 978-1-4624-0009-6 (sc)

Library of Congress Control Number: 2011938731

Printed in the United States of America

Inspiring Voices rev. date: 12/30/2011

DEDICATION

This book is dedicated to the memory of terminally ill patients, and the lives of patient families, who have benefited from the excellent, compassionate services of Hospice care, and to my dedicated colleagues and co-workers.

FROM: THE COMPLETE HOSPICE STAFF, made up of, Medical directors, Management, Nurses, Social Workers, Chaplains, Nurses' Aids, Home Health Aids, Secretaries, Bereavement Coordinators, Volunteer Coordinators and...

To: VOLUNTEERS THEMSELVES, who volunteer their effort, energy and time, to work without compensation or pay, and minister to patients who are imminently dying, and supportive families who so generously and unselfishly give the gift of attention and presence; *the gift of self.*

All of whom, going beyond the call of duty, have dedicated their lives to the care and treatment of the terminally ill during their end of life journey, consistent with the Biblical Golden Rule, i.e., *"Do unto others as you would have others do unto you,"* Matthew 7:12.

CONTENTS

PREFACE

DISCLAIMER:

It is neither the desire nor intent of the authors of this work, A Hospice Guide Book, Sub Title: *Hospice Care, A Wise Choice; Providing Quality Comfort Care through the End of Life's Journey,* to borrow from, or use without permission, words, phrases, or terms of others.

Rather, the intent is to set forth in clear, concise, straightforward, and unequivocal language, easily understood terms, phrases, and words which are generic to the Hospice industry but are *not* understood by the general public.

RANDOM SURVEY RESEARCH:

In a random survey blind study, conducted by the authors, 400 persons were questioned and asked: *"Do you know what the term Hospice means?"* 360 people answered *"No."* Not only did they *not* know *what* Hospice meant, neither had they ever *heard* the word.

This reflects an astonishing 80% *negative* response from those surveyed. Subsequently, the undeniable and *overwhelming* reason and purpose for writing this work, *A Hospice Guide Book*, becomes acutely obvious; to educate and enlighten the public at large by presenting an explanation in writing—all in one place—about *Hospice Care, A Wise Choice, emphasizing the important provision of comfort care through the end of life's journey* terminating in a comfortable, peaceful death with dignity.

There is much information about Hospice available on the internet—if you know where to look—however at best, the information provided is fragmented, and, at worst, it is presented on a Hospice Agency website directed toward soliciting Hospice patients for that particular agency.

Again, the *purpose* of this work is to place all Hospice information _ *in one location* _ at the fingertips of medical professionals, as well as lay persons. The *goal* is to definitively publish *A Hospice Guide Book* which can be effectively put to use by all.

Any material used in this publication presented as excerpts, quotes, or in full, are used with permission, or under Public Domain utilization from either Wikipedia, the free cyclopedia; North Central Florida Hospice, Inc. 1996, requesting to be credited thusly, "Please note: These articles are being made publicly available in the hope that they benefit others in the Hospice community. Feel free to use them provided you credit Hospice of North Central Florida with sole authorship and do not alter the content. Please include this note in any copies you choose to make."

Excerpts and quotes are also used with permission from another publication by the Author, Dr. Curtis E. Smith, titled, "*When It's Time*," PublishAmerica, Baltimore, 2008, et al articles, and publications which are credited in either the reference or resource sections.

All information in this publication A Hospice Guide Book is not intended as a substitute for information *about* Hospice Medical advice, and the reader should not take any action before consulting with a Hospice Professional and / or Medical doctors.

The contributing authors do not presume to speak on behalf of any *specific* Hospice agency, company or organization, as to setting down policies, procedures, methods, rules, standards, roles and/or responsibilities. Rather ___ *they present in part their testimony,* as a team member—*written from a third person perspective,* they share their role and responsibilities, in the broader sense, as *practicing, active* Hospice personnel speaking in *general terms,* with regard to *their* professional discipline and role, as viewed *by* them, *through their eyes.*

At the risk of being redundant, it is again stated, the purpose for writing and publishing this book is to educate, enlighten, and inform the general public about Hospice care. It is not intended to be inclusive, nor does it attempt to give medical advice.

Rather, the goal is to set down, all in one place, cogent available information about Hospice care in a clear, concise, understandable, and unambiguous way, thus, enabling the information to be understood by all.

If it satisfies that purpose, the effort, energy, and time spent researching and writing this work has been well rewarded, the purpose fulfilled, and the goal will have been met.

ACKNOWLEDGMENT

Many thanks to those who generously offered assistance in working with the author by answering questions, providing insight, and overall encouragement to challenge and inspire the research, compilation, and completion of this work.

The Interdisciplinary Group (IDG) team members, who have contributed their personal testimonies, and by so doing, have added a personal and professional touch to the contents. Their names appear alphabetically on the Credit page listed as Contributing Co-Authors.

A special thanks to my wife, Sandra, who sometimes watched me type pages of the manuscript, listened to me read aloud, and then personally read through each sentence, of every chapter, and made many invaluable contributions and suggestions.

To each of you, thanks, and God bless you.

CREDITS

Credit and recognition is hereby given to active participating team members, of an active Hospice agency organization, who have generously contributed to this work, A Hospice Guide Book; *Hospice Care, a Wise Choice.*

They have shared, and presented their personal testimonies, about memorable events which have occurred during their hospice career; experiences that have enriched and influenced their lives as a result of their interactions, and interventions with terminally ill Hospice patients.

They are listed in alphabetical order as co-authors.

Samina Arenas, Licensed Vocational Nurse (LVN)

Felix A. Colon, Rev., PHD. Chaplain

Valerie A. Cook, RN, AS, Patient Care Manager

June Diacon, Certified Home Health Aid (CHHA)

Judy Fawcett, Volunteer Coordinator

Susie Mendez, Admissions Coordinator

Betty Palao, Primary Care Giver

Trish Kulschar, Registered Nurse (RN) Patient Case Manager

Vivian Ro, MSW, Medical Social Worker

Bonnie Stead, Quality Control Manager

Gary Tucker, Rev., Bereavement Coordinator

INTRODUCTION

"A Hospice Guide Book" Subtitle, *"Hospice Care, A Wise Choice,"* is designed to educate and enlighten the general public about Hospice: its definition, its origin, its history, and modern day Hospice care.

As reported in the Preface, in a recent random, blind study survey, conducted by the author, 400 persons were questioned and asked: *"Do you know what the term Hospice means?"*360 people answered, *"No."* Not only did they *not know what* Hospice means, neither had they *ever heard* the word. This reflects an astonishing 80% uninformed, *negative* response from those surveyed.

Subsequently, the *undeniable* and *overwhelming* reason for publishing this work becomes acutely obvious; to educate and enlighten the public at large, about Hospice Care Benefits, by providing information, and by giving an overview explanation in writing—all in one place—about *Hospice Care.*

Thus, the work becomes *A Hospice Guide Book*; a valuable tool—that can be used by both professional and lay persons—i.e. professional Hospice and Medical employees, caregivers, and family members, describing and emphasizing the available and important benefit of *Hospice* (Medicaid) state financed, and (Medicare) a federal, publically funded programs which provide for *palliative care,* aka *comfort care,* through the patient's end-of-life's journey; terminating in a peaceful death; *death with dignity.*

PATIENT'S BILL OF RIGHTS

As a Hospice Patient, you have the Right:

To be informed and fully understand these rights and all the rules and regulations Governing patient conduct acknowledged by you, as a patient, or your representative prior to, or at the time of admission.

To be fully informed by a doctor of the patient's diagnosis and medical condition and be given the opportunity to participate or refuse to participate in the plan of care treatment, decision making, and to obtain complete, and current information regarding your health care status.

To receive pertinent information relating to advance directives, and applicable federal and state laws, and to be given assistance in completing same.

To be informed in advance of Hospice services to be provided, i.e. attending Physician, Registered Nurse (RN), Chaplain, Medical Social Worker, Volunteer, and Bereavement Counselor.

To be assured of confidential handling of clinical and medical records and prohibited unauthorized release of information to anyone other than those who have a right to know, i.e. law enforcement, insurance company's third-party payers.

To receive favorable expert healthcare without prejudice regarding race, religion, color, creed, marital status, sexual preference, sex, handicap, ager, or national origin, and to receive courteous and helpful understanding from hospice employees and staff.

To be fully informed of the medical procedures to be performed and risks involved to permit the patient to make informed intelligent decisions, or to refuse medical treatment.

To be able to facilitate and receive prompt treatment in emergency situations regardless of economic status.

PATIENT'S BILL OF RIGHTS

Each Hospice Patient or Family receiving Hospice Care has the Responsibility:

To read, understand, and sign the forms necessary for treatment:

To respect the rights and dignity of the healthcare providers, and to treat personnel with dignity and respect

To disclose medical information throughout the course of treatment and to cooperate with Hospice personnel

To be honest and direct in understanding the extent of patient illness and treatment and to accept the consequences for refusal of any medical treatment, and / or non-compliance

To inform the Hospice agency representative of any dissatisfaction with Hospice Care, and to be made aware of conditions of grievances, as explained by hospice personnel

To follow medical advice, treatment, and drug instructions, or to inform the Hospice provider agency of patient intent not to follow advice

To be home for scheduled appointments or to give cancellation notice to the Hospice provider agency 48 hours in advance of appointment

CHAPTER 1

WHAT IS HOSPICE?

a. History
b. Modern Day Hospice Care

History:

Hospice is more of a concept than a place for providing comfort for end-of-life care. According to the Wikipedia Free Encyclopedia the word "hospice" has its origin from the Latin word *hospes*. The original concept of Hospice was begun around the 11th century. Initially founded and dedicated as places to provide hospitality, care and treatment to the dying, incurably Ill, sick, or wounded, and was designed to serve as host to guests and cross-country travelers.

The Wikipedia Encyclopedia states that, "in the 14th century, the order of the Knights Hospitaller of St. John of Jerusalem opened the first hospice in Rhodes, meant to provide refuge for travelers, and care for the terminally ill and dying."

"In the United Kingdom, in the middle of the 19th century, greater emphasis was focused on the need for increased care and treatment of the terminally ill. By the year 1905 at least six hospices existed in England. About this same time the philosophy and development of hospice spread to Australia. From 1979 to 1907 three active hospice facilities had been established in Australia. The United State, in 1899, saw the opening of the first hospice, St. Rose's Hospice founded by the Servants for the Relief of Incurable Cancer. The concept was so successful that the organization soon opened facilities in six other cities.

1

"Some of the most influential advocates and early developers of hospice care Health facilities was the Irish Religious Sisters of Charity. Their work spread rapidly and they became an international organization.

"From 1890 until 1905 they opened hospice facilities in Sydney, Melbourne, and New South Wales. In 1905 they opened the St. Joseph Hospice in London. It was there that Cicely Saunders pioneered and developed many of the foundational principles of the modern day Hospice."

Modern Day Hospice Care

It was Dr. Cicely Saunders who pioneered, set forth, and developed many of the foundational principles of modern day Hospice Care. Dr. Saunders recognized death as a natural process. Her philosophy which encapsulates the Modern Day Hospice Philosophy, was neither to extend—by prolonging—nor hastening death. Rather, her philosophy and purpose was to provide physical, emotional, psychological social and spiritual care for the terminally ill patient in the comfort of their home, or in a home-like hospice facility setting enabling the patient to die a peaceful death with dignity.

A quote from Dr. Saunders appropriately expresses her philosophy about life, death and dying:

"…You matter to the last moment of your life,

And we will do all we can,

Not only to help you die peacefully,

*But also to live until you die."**

Dame Cicely Saunders
Founder of the Modern Day Hospice Movement

---

*Hospice neither prolongs the patient's life, nor hastens the patient's death.

CHAPTER 2

HOSPICE: FALLACIES, MYTHS, AND FACTS

For some, who think they have any knowledge about Hospice Care, there are many fallacies, myths, and misinterpretations. It is important to list common misunderstandings, fallacies, and myths, and at the same time to set the record straight, by listing relevant facts regarding Hospice.

To eliminate the misconceptions about hospice, it is extremely important to present the facts about Hospice—alongside the misunderstandings—in an attempt to educate the misinformed concerning Hospice Care, and eliminate the stigma attached to hospice.

Armed with the facts, and an enlightened sharing of them; attitudes will change, and more people who are diagnosed with a life-limiting, terminal Illness—and are found to be Hospice appropriate—will also become better informed, and more knowledgeable regarding the fallacies, myths, misinterpretations, and facts about Hospice Care.

Thus, enabling those who could become Hospice patients the opportunity to receive the benefit of expert comfort care, pain control management, symptom control, emotional, spiritual and psychosocial support, as they live with their terminal illness during the end-of-life stages, and peacefully transition from this life to the next.

Some of the fallacies, misinterpretations, and myths are listed as follows:

FALLACY: Hospice is a Place Where a Person Goes to Die:

FACT: Contrary to common belief, Hospice is not just a place to go to die. Hospice is more of a concept rather than a *place*.

Hospice, provided primarily in the home with a Primary Caregiver (PCG), is designed and planned to offer compassionate comfort care to terminally ill patients who have been diagnosed with a life expectancy to live, 6 months or less.

FALLACY: Hospice Means Losing Hope:

FACT: Because the patient is imminently dying, choosing Hospice care does not mean the individual is losing hope. Far from it; it means re-establishing priorities. Whereas, prior to becoming a Hospice patient there was hope for healing, the patient now has a realistic hope of living in the comfort of their own home, surrounded by loved ones, experiencing a comfortable quality of life, with needs met, free-from-pain,

FALLACY: Hospice is Only for Patients That Are Going to Die Quickly:

FACT: This is simply not true. Often times when a patient is admitted to Hospice, and they begin to receive appropriate medical care, plus the multiple sources of compassionate, and supportive care provided by Interdisciplinary Group (IDG) members, many respond positively and frequently live beyond the diagnosed 6 month life expectancy.

FALLACY: Hospice is Only for Cancer Patients:

FACT: This is false; statistics show that 50 plus percent (50%) of Hospice patients have a non-cancerous disease diagnosis. Whether or not the disease is cancer, the Interdisciplinary Group (IDG) team of professionals is qualified and skilled at managing symptoms of cancer and other terminal illnesses.

FALLACY: As a Hospice Patient will I Have to Sign a Do Not Resuscitate (DNR) Form

FACT: It is not a requirement to have a DNR agreement in place at the time of admission to Hospice. When a patient signs a DNR it is to advise the medical treatment staff that they do not want to be resuscitated if they stop breathing (Respiratory Distress), have a heart attack (stroke) aka CVA (Cardiovascular Attack), or the heart stops (Cardiac Arrest).

Hospice providers follow the choice and will of the patient and family. The goal of Hospice is to provide the patient with quality comfort care, and to help them maintain a level of independence by directing their own care.

CHAPTER 3

THE HOSPICE PHILOSOPHY

THE HOSPICE PHILOSOPHY

Modern day Hospice philosophy flies in the face of *euthanasia*, that is, the patient making a decision to take their own life via medication prescribed by a physician.

The majority of people want their loved to live as long, as possible, even with an incurable disease. However, there comes a time when aggressive treatment of the loved one's disease is no longer appropriate, and may encourage them to decide that the burden exceeds the realistic benefit. This validates their freedom to choose the best quality of life possible, for whatever length of life; Hospice Care.

When a patient's disease has reached an incurable point, the medical modality of treatment changes, from *curative* care to *palliative* (comfort) care. Under palliative care a range of treatments for symptoms may continue, including *chemotherapy, radiation, blood transfusions, paracentesis* (withdrawing fluid from the body, usually the abdomen), and *tube feeding*.

These are all considered to be medical *comfort measures*; to achieve comfort care, and to relieve the pain.

When the decision is reached to discontinue curative care, i.e., the medical model of Treatment, attempting to *treat and cure the disease*, moves to treating *the patient with a palliative modality*. That is, to provide comfort care, and to relieve pain, for as long as the patient has left to live.

The Hospice Benefit Program movement is designed to avoid prolonging suffering from ineffective medical efforts to conquer death, as opposed to the opposite extreme, ignoring the patient's approaching imminent death; ignoring the dying, is not a modern concept.

The culture of accepting the inevitable, in order to focus on easing the pathway from one phase of life to another, has deep roots extending back centuries, and even millennia, to periods when devoted spiritual leaders provided nurturing refuge to those in need, with the thought that God loves every person, and with the concept that Hospice Care is a worthwhile means for caregivers to return this love.

The ancient Hospice tradition has now been revived in the modern Hospice movement, in which, caring for the dying is not considered to be *a burden*, rather, *an opportunity* to provide comfort care with love, and enables a less difficult transition from this world to the next.

Revival of the modern Hospice concept came to fruition during the cultural turmoil of the 1960's, at which time Dr. Cicely Saunders pioneered and defined a Hospice program in 1968 at the Christopher's Hospital in London, England. The following year Dr. Elisabeth Kubler-Ross was a pioneer working with death and dying, and published a renowned work on *Death and Dying in America*.

The profound teachings and work of both Dr. Elisabeth Kubler-Ross, and Dr. Cicely Saunders throughout their active professional lives caused greater insight into both the pathway to death, and dying. Their work and concept is best expressed in the words of Dr. Cicely Saunders: *"The community needs the dying to make it think of eternal issues. We are indebted those who can make us learn such things as to be gentle and to approach others with true affection and respect."*

It appears as if she had returned full circle to the original concept of Hospice that has existed in all cultures since the beginning of human life.

Today, the revived concept and practice of Hospice Care provides a new, holistic discipline and is a permanent part of modern life; it is an important response to ever changing cultural conditions.

The distinct purpose of Hospice is to provide appropriate care and comfort, and a 24 Hour availability of professional care giver team members, who are sensitive to the patient's needs, enabling the patient to be remain in familiar surroundings, so as to better prepare the patient mentally, physically and spiritually for the major transition from this life to the next.[1]

Certification by a physician of a patient to Hospice care is based on the patient proximity to death, i.e. a life expectancy of 6 months or less.

Prior to acceptance, and admission, of a patient into a Hospice program the patient must sign a statement requesting Hospice care.

As previously stated, Hospice provides comfort care through the end of life's journey; Hospice neither prolongs the life, nor hastens the hospice patient's death.

In the Preface of this work, under *Survey Research*, the following information was stated in a random blind survey study, conducted by the authors, 400 persons were questioned and asked: *"Do you know what the term Hospice means?"* 360 people answered *"No."* Not only did they *not know what* Hospice *meant*; neither had they ever *heard* the word. This reflects an astonishing 80% *negative response* from those surveyed.

Subsequently, the undeniable and *overwhelming* reason and purpose for writing this work, A Hospice Guide Book, becomes acutely obvious; to educate the public at large by providing an explanation in writing—all in one place—with a Hospice Guide Book *emphasizing the important provision of comfort care through the end of life journey*; a peaceful death with dignity.

Therefore, it is extremely important to present the facts about Hospice—alongside the misunderstandings—in an attempt to educate the misinformed concerning Hospice care, and eliminate the stigma attached to Hospice. The Fallacies and Myths vs. Facts are set forth herein.

Armed with the facts, is hoped that there will be a sharing of them, that attitudes will change, and that more people who are diagnosed with a life-limiting Terminal Illness, and are Hospice appropriate, will also become better informed, and more knowledgeable regarding the fallacies, myths and facts about Hospice Care.

Thus, enabling those who could become Hospice patients the opportunity to receive the benefit of expert comfort care, pain control management, symptom control, emotional, spiritual and psychosocial support, as they live with their terminal illness, during the end-of-life stages, and have a peaceful transition from this life to the next.

CHAPTER 4

TERMINAL DIAGNOSIS:

a. **Common Diagnosis—(See Diagnosis List)**
b. **Uncommon Diagnosis**
c. **Definitions of Hospice Diagnosis; Eligibility and Medical Terms**

TERMINAL DISEASES

Medicare publishes guidelines which specify diseases that qualify for Hospice as terminal.

In order to qualify for Medicare Hospice coverage the diagnosis has to be certified by two medical doctors ___ usually the patient's primary care, or attending, physician and the Hospice medical director ___ confirming that the prospective patient has one or more terminal diseases, or else qualifies under the non-specific category designated as "failure to thrive."

The most common and debilitating are metastatic cancer, (which, at the time of this writing represented more than fifty percent of all hospice patients); irreparable organ failure, such as decompensated cirrhosis of the liver; uremia (renal failure) not amenable to dialysis; Stage IV Congestive Heart Failure (CHF); irreversible respiratory failure; sepsis (destruction of tissue by bacterial toxins), and anoxic encephalopathy.

Modern medicine, medical research, life support equipment, and technology *can postpone* the onset of death, but cannot cure the terminal disease, notwithstanding the challenges and opportunities presented by advanced technology.

Patients with a life-limiting terminal illness, in fact, often receive little or no benefit from such medical treatments; and the treatments may increase the burden of living. For instance, such treatments may only extend the symptoms of the underlying disease.

Palliative care can alleviate the symptoms exhibited by these terminal illnesses. The most common symptoms are: dyspnea (painful and labored breathing); respiratory secretions; dysphagia (difficulty in swallowing); cough; painful hiccups; nausea, vomiting; cachexia (word pronounced: ka-keks-e-a—dehydration and emaciation); constipation; diarrhea; bowel obstruction; pruritis (skin inflammation); neuropathy (nerve pain); fatigue, anxiety; severe depression; delirium, and combinations of these symptoms.

THE MOST COMMON DISEASES

- Cancer

- Stroke

- Acute Cerebrovascular Accident (CVA)

- Dementia

- Alzheimer's Dementia
- Cardiac Disease
- Heart Disease Congestive Heart Failure (CHF)
- Pulmonary Disease
- Chronic Obstructive Pulmonary Disease (COPD)
- Emphysema
- Liver Disease (Cirrhosis , primary)
- Renal Disease (Kidney Failure)
- AIDS (Acquired Immune Deficiency Disease)
- Amyotrophic Schlerosis (ALS)
- Failure to Thrive (FTT)

LESS COMMON DISEASES

* Huntington's' Chorea

* Paralysis Agitans aka (Parkinson's Disease)

* Joint Osteoporosis

* Intracranial Hemorrhage (caused by rupture of an aneurysm)

* Senile Degenerate Brain

* Anemia

DEFINITIONS OF HOSPICE DIAGNOSIS ELIGIBILITY AND MEDICAL TERMS: <u>Listed in Order of Commonality</u>

NOTE: While these terms are primarily hospice specific they are not intended to be inclusive, diagnostic, or medically definitive, nor intended to give medical advice. The intended purpose is to present only a *brief overview*, and a *general broad description* of various diseases. Any patient, or any other persons seeking medical advice, or definitive diagnoses, should consult and confer with their own medical doctor.

CANCER: CA Cancer is an invasion of tissues by a growth of abnormal malignant cells. A cell divides and reproduces abnormally with uncontrolled growth and often spreads (*metastasize*) to other sites in the body. The exact cause of cancer is unknown, however, most forms of cancer can be traced to precipitating factors such as, cigarette, pipe, cigar smoking, overexposure to the sun, exposure to cancer causing chemicals called carcinogens; ionizing radiation; it is believed that viruses are associated with some types of cancer. Cancer is not contagious, and neither can it be inherited, however, genetic (*familial*) tendency susceptibility plays a role in certain forms of the disease.

Types of Cancer: Different types of cancer vary greatly with age, ethnic group, geographical location and sex. According to statistics, in the United States, heart disease is the leading cause of death; cancer is the second cause of death, with breast cancer and lung cancer identified as leading the statistics.

Probability of Getting: At age 25 the probability of developing cancer within 5 years is 1 in 700; however, the older population is much more prone to cancer: for the older persons at age 65 the probability of developing cancer within 5 years, is 1 in 14.

Anatomy Parts Most Affected: The parts of the body most affected by cancer are the breasts; bone marrow, oral cavity, colon; lungs; prostate, and uterus.

Signs of Cancer: Signs of cancer include a change in bladder or bowel habits; a sore that won't heal; a persistent cough or hoarseness; indigestion or difficulty in swallowing; unusual bleeding or discharge; thickening or lump in the breast or other part of the body; change in a wart or mole, and unexplained loss of weight.

Treatment: The prognosis depends on the type and site of the cancer, and the promptness of initial treatment. Cancer may involve surgery, and/or, chemotherapy and radiation...

Probability of Cure: Statistics reveal that approximately one-third of newly diagnosed cancer patients are permanently cured with early detection diagnosis and prompt initial treatment.

When the Cancer spreads *(metastasizes)* to an inoperable and incurable state it is then considered to be Hospice Appropriate: For example, Cancer can be diagnosed as Hospice Appropriate when the disease does not respond to curative medical treatment, and exacerbates through metastasizing to other organs, causing the body to become compromised and weakened exhibiting casual signs and symptoms.

STROKE: (See Cerebrovascular accident (CVA)

CEREBROVASCULAR ACCIDENT (CVA): Oxygen deprivation or starvation caused by an abnormal condition in which hemorrhage or blockage of the blood vessels of the brain leads to resulting symptoms, e.g., sudden loss of ability to move a body part (as an arm, leg or the face) or to speak. Paralysis; weakness; or if severe, can result in death. Usually, only one side of the body is affected.

DEMENTIA: A progressive state of mental decline, especially of memory function and judgment. When it is caused by Alzheimer's disease, brain injury or by degeneration brought about by aging (senile dementia), changes that occur are irreversible.

The mental decline is often accompanied by disorientation, stupor, and disintegration of the personality

ALZHEIMER'S DISEASE: A common disorder affecting both men and women, it usually starts between ages 50 and 60, often with memory lapses and changes in behavior. Its primary symptom progression is loss of short-term memory, mental ability and function; it is often accompanied by personality changes and emotional instability. The disease progresses to include symptoms of confusion, restlessness, inability to plan and carry out activities, delusional behavior, sometimes hallucinations and loss of sphincter (i.e., bladder) control. The cause is unknown but plaques and neurofibrillary tangles are commonly found in the brain tissues. There is no cure; treatment is aimed at alleviating and reducing the symptoms.

CARDIAC (Heart) DISEASE: Any identified disease pertaining to the heart causing a cardiac condition disorder; a disease of the heart resulting in damage to the heart such as, coronary artery disease (CAD), and cardiomyopathy. Cardiomyopathy, is a primary disease of the muscles of the heart, and causes range from congenital (from birth) factors to viral infection, to coronary artery disease.

(CHF) CONGESTIVE HEART FAILURE: This disease is usually caused by a heart disorder and often develops chronically with shortness of breath, due to fluid accumulation in the lungs, and edema (swelling) of the extremities. The disease symptoms is identified as an abnormal condition characterized by circulatory congestion, and retention of salt and water by the kidneys; it is usually caused by a heart disorder

PULMONARY DISEASE: The term Pulmonary refers to the lungs or respiratory system. The disease range can affect: pulmonary artery; pulmonary circulation; pulmonary edema; and pulmonary embolism (blockage of a blood vessel, especially an artery.

(COPD) CHRONIC OBSTRUCTIVE PULMONARY DISEASE: A general term identifying chronic, or terminal irreversible lung disease and is usually a combination of emphysema and chronic bronchitis. COPD patients often have been, or are, heavy smokers.

EMPHYSEMA: This is an abnormal condition of the lungs in which there is over inflation of the air sacs (alveoli) of the lungs, leading to a breakdown of their walls, a decrease in respiratory function, and, in severe cases, increasing breathlessness.

Severe case may require oxygen.

LIVER DISEASE (Cirrhosis; Primary): This is a chronic disease condition of the liver in which fibrous tissue and nodules replace normal tissue, interfering with blood flow and normal functions of the organ, including, gastrointestinal functions, hormone metabolism, alcohol and drug detoxification. The major cause of cirrhosis is chronic alcoholism. If untreated, liver and kidney failure and gastrointestinal hemorrhage can occur, leading to death.

END-STAGE RENAL DISEASE (Kidney—Renal Failure): The instability of the kidney to excrete wastes and function in the maintenance of the electrolyte balance. Acute renal failure is characterized by inability to produce urine and an accumulation of wastes, is often associated with trauma, burns, acute infection, or obstruction of the urinary tract. If untreated, acute kidney failure can occur, leading to death.

AIDS: (Acquired Immune Deficiency disease): This is a serious, often fatal, condition in which the immune system breaks down and does not respond normally to infection. The victims often develop Kaposi's sarcoma, and recurrent severe infections. The cause has been identified as a virus (human immunodeficiency virus (HIV). No current treatment has yet proven effective.

(ALS) AMYOTROPHIC SCHLEROSIS:

Sometimes referred to as: CNS (Central Nervous System Disease) A degenerative disease of the central nervous system characterized by progressive muscle atrophy starting in the limbs and spreading to the rest of the body, often accompanied by hyperreflexia (overactive reflexes). There is no known cause for the disease, and usually manifests itself after age 40 affecting more men than women; the disease progresses rapidly. There is no known cure or treatment; also called Lou Gehrig's disease.

(FTT) FAILURE TO THRIVE: FTT is used to designate a symptom often occurring in patients with a variety of acute illnesses that are known to interfere with normal nutrient intake, absorption, metabolism, or excretion, or to result in greater-than-normal energy requirements, resulting in a terminal diagnosis of FTT for acute irreversible malnutrition.

HUNTINGTON'S' CHOREA: An abnormal hereditary condition (autosomal dominant disease) characterized by progressive chorea (involuntary rapid, jerky motions) and mental deterioration, leading to dementia. Symptoms usually appear in the third or fourth decade of life and progress to death, often within 15 years.

PARALYSIS AGITANS aka *(***Parkinson's Disease***):* A slowly progressive neurological disorder characterized by resting tremor, shuffling gait, stooped posture, rolling motion of the fingers, drooling, and muscle weakness, sometimes with emotional instability. Occurring usually after age 60, and then, its cause is unknown; but it may also occur in young persons as a result of encephalitis, syphilis, or certain other diseases.

JOINT OSTEOPOROSIS: The abnormal loss of boney tissue causing fragile bones, that fracture easily, accompanied by acute pain, especially in the back; and loss of stature.

It can cause abnormal loss of boney tissue and irreversible damage which could result in a terminal diagnosis causing death.

INTRACRANIAL ANEURYSM HEMORRHAGE (caused by rupture of an aneurysm): Aneurysm of a cranial artery. Symptoms include headache, stiff neck, nausea, and sometimes loss of consciousness; rupture of an aneurysm is a serious, and often fatal, condition.

END-STAGE SENILE DEGENERATE BRAIN; (AKA senile dementia): A mental disorder of the aged, resulting from atrophy and degeneration of the brain, with no sign of cerebrovascular disease. Symptoms, which are usually progressive, include loss of memory, periods of confusion and irritability, confabulation (invention of fictious details about a past event that may or may not have occurred), and poor judgment.

ANEMIA: A condition in which the hemoglobin content of the blood is below normal limits. It is the result of a defect in the production of hemoglobin, and its carrier, the red blood cells. The most common cause is a deficiency in iron, an element necessary for the formation of hemoglobin. There are several types of anemia, including aplastic, pernicious, sickle cell, and thalassemia.

CHAPTER 5

ALTERNATIVE MEDICAL
CARE MODALITIES

a. **CURATIVE: Aggressive Medical Treatment**
b. **PALLIATIVE: Hospice Care**
c. **A HOLISTIC Approach**
d. **A "DO NOTHING" Approach**

Curative Care:

Curative Care is also known as Aggressive Medical Care Treatment. It can be defined as: A Medical science technology measure used with a patient when there is a belief that the patient will recover, will eventually get well, or that will prolong the life of the patient with an acceptable quality.

When a patient chooses to receive Curative Care, aka Aggressive Medical Care treatment, they will receive every known medical science modality and technique for treatment, such as antibiotics for infections, chemotherapy, and radiation for cancer, dialysis for renal failure, or surgery, and any other medical interventions available that is designed to preserve or prolong life to treat the disease or illness

When the disease or illness does not respond positively to any of the medical treatments the attending physician may use sensitivity to guide the patient and/or family away from seeking aggressive medical treatment to save the patient's life to seeing the value end-of-life care palliative aka comfort care. Palliative care will be defined and discussed here in the next section, and also re-stated in Chapter 6, under the heading, Levels of Hospice Care / Treatments.

Sometimes patients and families will not accept the reality of curative medicine being ineffective, even to the point of going to court to try and force the medical providers to comply with continued aggressive treatment.

Patients with strong religious beliefs may even turn to an exorcism for healing; (Origin: Late Latin, from Greek exorkizein-to bind by oath). Exorcism is the practice of evicting demons or other spiritual entities from a person or place which they are believed to have possessed by causing the entity to swear an oath. The practice is quite ancient and part of the belief system of many cultures.

Notwithstanding the fact that the practice is ancient, and an unproved certainty for healing, it is rare, but there are those willing to use any means to effect healing even if it means resorting to nontraditional, unorthodox and radical behavior.

Palliative Care

Palliative Care focuses on making the end of life journey as comfortable and worthwhile for the Hospice patient. It provide a peace of mind that is reinforced by monitored medication and symptom control 24 hours a day, 7 days a week, with medical attention only a phone call away.

The Hospice Benefits Program delivers quality and compassionate care to patients who are facing a shortened life span due to a terminal illness diagnosis. The overall hospice and palliative care—by making available professional counseling support—enables the patient to deal with emotional and spiritual issues. The Hospice Benefits Program is customized to the patient's individual medical, psychosocial, social, emotional, and spiritual needs.

Palliative Care zeros in and focuses on reducing the level of pain, and the severity of symptoms of the terminal illness, rather than attempting to provide a cure. The goal is to make the patient as comfortable as possible, providing enhanced quality of life to include, medical emotional, psychosocial, psychological, and spiritual needs for whatever remaining time the patient has.

Hospice Care makes it possible for a patient, with a life-limiting illness, to face each day surrounded by loving, compassionate care, and live for whatever life remains, with loving attention, a sense of serenity, and to die a peaceful death with dignity.

A Holistic Care Approach

Holistic Medicine has been practiced by hundreds of thousands, perhaps millions, of people around the world. Holistic Medicine attempts to address the whole person, i.e., body, mind, spirit, and emotions.

After having tried every modality of Medical Treatment without success, many living with a Terminal Illness diagnosis would choose to use a nontraditional and unorthodox modality of treatment with Holistic Medicine. The use of Holistic Medicine relies on attempts to restore balance to the entire body system of the person with nutrition, herbal supplements, bio-identical hormones and homeopathy to include attempts to restore the body's healing power resource with osteopathic manipulation.

There are those terminally ill patients who have chosen to use Holistic Medicine as an alternative method for healing become persuaded that the Holistic Medicine approach is a route to a "Silver Bullet cure." In so doing they perpetually look for a "magic' herb or macro-nutrient supplement as a primary method for their Holistic Medicine treatment.

While minimal benefits may be obtained from such treatment, the limited success may be followed by periods of little or no measurable progress. There is a danger to the patient in relying on these type of Holistic Medicine treatments; medical science proves that they rarely, if ever, cure or heal the illness but can instead, temporarily delay or suppress the disease symptoms, and in the long term, be a causative factor for more serious health condition side effects.

Some terminally ill patients become so obsessed with being cured or getting well that they lose touch with reality and cling to unrealistic expectations.

Holistic Medicine Summary: There is a caution for anyone with a life-limiting terminal illness electing to use Holistic Medicine as an alternative for medically approved and recognized methods and procedures for treatment.

The terminally ill patient, who is considering the use of Alternative Medicine, would be wise to carefully examine the methodology that a Holistic Medical practioner is suggesting for use. Especially with regard to potential benefits weighed against side-effects, and any written history attesting to success of use, along with realistic expectation for relief or cure, the expected duration of treatments, and last but certainly not least, the anticipated costs involved.

Be aware that most health plans do not cover Alternative Holistic Medicine costs for patient treatment with herbs, and nutrients; it will be an out-of-pocket expense for the patient.

A final caution: *"Buyer beware."*

A "Do Nothing" Approach:

There are those, when diagnosed with a terminal illness, that doesn't want any type of care or treatment. Choosing instead to, in their own words: *"Just let me die in peace."*

Not to make a choice, is to make a choice.

Every patient, terminally ill or sustaining other disease symptoms, has the right, under "Patient's Rights," to choose the plan of care for their life.

Sometimes, family members try and persuade loved ones' who have made a decision not to seek care or treatment, to change their mind.

While the family may believe they are acting in the best interest of the patient, the patient's choice must take precedence.

In the event hospice medical personnel are contacted, and asked to try to get the patient to change their mind, to not seek medical care or treatment, the medical personnel will refuse.

Neither will the medical professional attempt to intervene in any way to try and persuade patients to change their decision, to not seek medical care or treatment.

It would be both ethically, morally, and legally wrong to try and interfere with a patient's rights.

As difficult as it may be for family members to observe a loved one slowly decline and imminently die; the patient's wishes necessarily need to be honored in all cases.

Again, at the risk of being redundant, the patient's choice and wishes take precedence, and *must* be honored at all times.

That's how it is; *it is what it is.*

CHAPTER 6

THE HOSPICE TEAM: ROLE AND RESPONSIBILITIES

a. MD Medical Director
b. Admissions Coordinator
c. Patient Care Manager (PCM)
d. RN Case Manager
e. MSW Medical Social Worker (SW)
f. Clergy—Chaplain for Spiritual Care (SCC)
g. CHHA—Home Health Aid
h. Bereavement Coordinator (BC)
i. Volunteer Coordinator (VC)
j. Primary Care Giver (PCG)
k. CQI—Continuing Quality Improvement Manager

This Hospice Guide Book provides a brief description for the role and responsibility of each hospice component Interdisciplinary Group Members.

Medical Director: MD

Each hospice agency program has a Medical Director. Federal Law 42 CFR418.54 sets forth the controlling regulations: It states the Medical Director, *"Assumes overall responsibility for the medical component of the hospice's patient care program."*

Thus, this is the role of the Medical Director, but is not limited to simply assuming the "overall, responsibility."

They are responsible for the medical management of the hospice patient's treatment and plan of care (POC) for the duration of the patient's length of stay in the Hospice program.

Additionally, the Medical Director oversees ongoing medical services and coordinates care from other providers including the patient's Primary Physician aka Attending Physician.

The Medical Director confirms the terminal diagnosis certification with the Attending Physician aka Primary Physician, and the patient's prognosis (estimated duration of illness) of six (6) months or less. They attend and monitor all Interdisciplinary Group (IDG) meetings and review the team's Plan of Care (POC) for each patient.

To ensure that each and every patient receives the best, most appropriate, needed and necessary medical care available. In addition, they review all patient medical charts and monitor the Registered Nurse (RN) Case Manager Treatment modalities, and patient's ongoing physical condition.

This is accomplished to determine that the patient is continuing in a slow decline with weight loss, decreased strength, decreased verbalization, and decreased energy, and continues to be appropriate for hospice care and support, and without hospice care their condition would rapidly exacerbate (get worse).

Admissions Coordinator

The Admissions Coordinator

The hospice Admissions Coordinator is usually the first point of contact following a patient referral.

The Admissions Coordinator assumes primary responsibility for admitting patients into a Hospice program. And subsequently, informing the patient that they are giving up the right to aggressive treatment when entering the Hospice Care program.

Patient confidentiality is a very important dynamic and is rigidly enforced through state Laws, and federal regulations known as the Health Insurance Accountability Act (HIPPA) 1996, i.e., HIPPA

Policy 6.1. Violations are legally and stringently enforced with stringent penalties, imposed by both civil and criminal courts.

The Admissions Coordinator duties include, but are not limited to: Assuring patient confidentiality and to identity that the following specific patient information is collected and verified prior to admitting a patient into a hospice program:

Name	Diagnosis
Age	Medical History
Address	Medications
Social Security #	Health Status

Patient confidentiality and privacy is a very important dynamic in health care management and is rigidly enforced through state and federal regulations known as the Health Insurance Portability and Accountability Act (HIPPA) passed by Congress 1996. Strict laws are in place to protect patient privacy and confidentiality; HIPPA Policy 6.1. Violations are legally and stringently enforced, by both civil and criminal courts, with heavy monetary penalties, and possible imprisonment.

Additionally, the Admissions Coordinator collects and verifies appropriate patient Medical History performs the following duties:

- Informs the patient that they are giving up the right to aggressive treatment when entering the Hospice Care program
- Obtains necessary information to support the physician's referral prior to setting an Appointment for an Explanation of Benefits (EOB).
- Contacts the patient or family to schedule an appointment for an Explanation of Benefits (EOB) within 24 hours after receiving the referral.
- Obtain the referral diagnosis and, prognosis (six (6) months or less of life
- (Expectancy) and, pertinent data that support the terminal diagnosis.

- Obtain information on physician's orders for medications, treatments, and symptom management, as well as any information about the medical management of patient conditions that are not related to the terminal diagnosis.
- These are usually accompanying physical ailment disease indicators which are commonly referred to in the medical field as *comorbidities* and are defined as: two or more coexisting medical conditions or diseases processes that are in addition to the initial diagnosis.
- In a timely manner, request a Discharge Summary Order be obtained from any medical facility, e.g. hospital, or health care facility, e.g. Skilled Nursing Facility, from which the patient has recently been discharged.
- Obtain patient dietary and nutrition information including any diet restrictions.
- Assures patient and family of confidentiality regarding patient history and Medical records
- Inform patient about the importance of having a Primary Care Giver
- Inform about Policies relating to patient living alone, etc.
- Assure patient of hospice 24 Hour 7 day week availability. De-emphasize 911 calls by informing patient that, they are giving up rights to aggressive care, with regard to treatment for their Terminal Illness, when they voluntarily choose to become a Hospice patient

NOTE: There are certain other legal documents and other information which will be requested from a patient at the time of admission when they enroll as a Hospice patient. These documents and additional information include the following:

An Advance Directive

A Durable Power of Attorney for Health purposes

A General Durable Power of Attorney for Finances / Real Estate transactions (suggested)

Assignment of a Primary Caregiver (suggested)

A Living Will (suggested)

Funeral arrangement plans as to mortuary.

A Do Not Resuscitate Form (suggested—not necessary for admission). The DNR is a legal document form stating that the patient has voluntarily chosen hospice care, is aware of approaching death, and understands in doing so has given up the option to seek curative, aggressive treatment.

The *required* legal documents will be briefly discussed. The Medical Social will be able to discuss with the patient and family the importance of each legal document required as well as the importance of the suggested information.

Advance Directive aka Living Will: There are two kinds of documents; Medical (Durable) Power of Attorney, and Living Wills. Provides direction to surrogates about future medical treatment wanted in case of patient incapacity. An Advance Directive or Living Will allows an individual while still living and cognitive to document their wishes concerning medical care and treatment at the end of their life. See Also Appendage for **POLST** Reference

Durable Power of Attorney (Health): A legal document designating another person to make health decisions for the patient if the patient is incapacitated and unable to make decisions for themselves.

Durable Power of Attorney (General): A general Power of Attorney is used to allow an appointed agent all business, financial, legal, or other affairs during a period of time when the individual / patient is incapacitated and unable to do so.

A Testimony of an Active Practicing Admissions Coordinator

My name is Susie Mendez. I am an Admissions Coordinator for a major Hospice Agency in Southern California where I have worked for over 3 years. My background and education is in the medical field as a Pharmacy Technician. Until I begin working with hospice my medical knowledge outside the pharmacy field was limited. My reason for changing positions was to widen my horizons; to expand and increase my medical knowledge and education.

From a friend I heard of an employment opportunity for an Admission Coordinator position with a large national Hospice Agency. I subsequently applied for the position and was hired.

As a member of the hospice team I soon became familiar with the hospice care Benefits Program and how to explain it to others. I was then, and am now, impressed with the thoughtful caring concept, upon which the origin of hospice was founded, i.e., providing compassionate care to those dying from a terminal illness; what a wonderful program!

My responsibility is to accept referrals from physicians, nurses, social workers, chaplains, hospitals, health care agencies, and the community at large.

My specific duties include, but are not limited to: Assuring patient privacy, and patient Confidentiality, and make sure the following information is collected and verified prior to admitting a patient into the hospice program:

Full Name; Date of Birth; Social Security Number; Medicare ID / Insurance Card ID, and to explain hospice benefits to patients and family members, about what hospice is, and what the program can provide for the patient and the family.

The more involved I become in admitting patients to the hospice care program the more I enjoy and love my work.

I thoroughly love the opportunity to explain and share, with prospective patients and their families, information about the end-of-life benefits available to them.

It is rewarding, and makes me feel good, as the benefits are explained I often sense both the patient's and family's level of anxiety and hopelessness is lessened.

In my work the most pleasant experience comes when patient and family are able to face the reality of imminent death and, at the same time, increase their knowledge as they learn about the dynamics of end-of-life care, and death and dying.

As I said, the more involved I become, in admitting patients to the hospice care program, the more I like and enjoy my work. My position is truly a work of caring, compassion, and love.

In some small way, I like to believe I am helping, especially the patient, as well as the family, to be able to cope more appropriately— during this very difficult and painful time—while they learn about how hospice care can help their loved one be able to move through the stages of death and dying, to imminently die a peaceful death, with dignity.

My name is Susie Mendez; this is my Personal Testimony and I approve of it being published.

The Start of Care aka Admission

Following the Explanation of Benefit appointment the patient may, at that time, request Hospice services.

If this is the patient and family's desire the patient can sign a statement requesting hospice care and can be admitted to service within a reasonable time, usually within a 24 hour period.

When a patient voluntarily requests to be entered into a hospice program, at the time of admission, the hospice personnel conducting the patient admission Start of Care (SOC)—usually a Registered Nurse (RN)—will ensure that the patient and family are fully informed concerning hospice benefits including, but not limited to:

1. Obtaining patient permission for the Consent of Care and Assignment of Benefits
2. Form to be signed, to include the Release of Information and Medical Records Form, with regard to patient care. Again, at this time, the importance of Patient information confidentiality needs to be emphasized
3. Fully explain the scope of hospice services to be provided including the entire
   Interdisciplinary Team support, Bereavement and Volunteer services
4. Hospice Requirement for a Durable Power of Attorney for Health Care Decisions
5. A Do Not Resuscitate Form—if appropriate
6. Provide a Patient' Right and Responsibility Form
7. Complete Medicare Benefits—Patient and Family Information
8. Complete patient Initial Nursing Assessment (INA) Form. The INA can be completed by the RN who is bringing the patient on to service, at the Start of Care (SOC), i.e., time of admission

Determining Number of Patient Care Managers (PCM)

The size of the census for the Hospice Agency usually determines the structure level for management.

Most agencies divide the total census into teams. For each team there is an identified team called the Interdisciplinary Health Care Group (IDG) assigned, consisting of but not limited to professional members as follows.

The Hospice Team:

a. **MD Medical Director**
b. **Patient Care Manager (PCM)**
c. **Registered Nurse (RN) Case Manager**
d. **Medical Social Worker (MSW)**
e. **Clergy—Chaplain for Spiritual Care (SCC)**
f. **CHHA—Certified Home Health Aid**
g. **Volunteer, if appropriate, and requested by patient/ family**

Although each team has specific Interdisciplinary assigned members, there is designated components which provide services to all teams, and to the overall hospice program.

They are:
Bereavement Coordinator (BC)

Volunteer Coordinator (VC)

CQI—Continuing Quality Improvement Manager

Patient Care Manager (PCM) R.N.

The Patient Care Manager (PCM) duties and responsibilities include, but are not limited to the following:

The Interdisciplinary Group (IDG) is led by the Patient Care Manager (PCM) who is responsible for coordinating all of the patient's service, and Plan of Care (POC), from the admission start of (SOC) to the patient's death, or other type discharge.

The Patient Care Manager (PCM) attends all Interdisciplinary Group (IDG) meetings and communicates on a regular basis with the patient, and the Registered Nurse (RN) Case Manager, providing a direct link between them, enabling clear communication to freely flow, permitting the exchange of patient information helping them to stay informed about the patient's clinical and medical condition.

Both also maintain an "as needed" direct contact with the Medical Director, and pharmacists, to be able to obtain the physician orders and, to obtain the necessary authorization for pain medication, and other medications, plus dieticians, and all other members of the Health Care Team, for ongoing patient care and comfort needs.

Realistically, every patient's Plan of Care (POC) details a program of care and services to be provided, ensuring the patient and family members will be receive customized, excellent care for the patient's best possible quality of life, for whatever length of life remains.

A Testimony of an Active Practicing R.N. Patient Care Manager (PCM)

My name is Valerie Cook, RN, PCM. I am a Patient Care Manger for a National Hospice Organization in Southern California. I received my nursing education at Mt. San Antonio College, graduating with an R.N. and A.S. Degree. I have been a Registered Nurse (RN) for many years and a Hospice Patient Care Manager for several.

The reason I chose Hospice is because of my father. I live in Southern California; my father and mother lived 400 miles away in Northern California. In 2004 my father was experiencing a debilitating disease. In 2004 he was diagnosed with mesothelioma, a terminal illness. Always a fighter he fought the life-limiting condition until it became obvious he was losing the battle. His doctor recommended hospice, and in June 2005.he signed onto a local hospice program.

Almost immediately the hospice Interdisciplinary Group (IDG) team came into the home. They appeared to be miraculous; they took charge of his condition, managed his case, and controlled his symptoms, with compassionate care and professional skill.

All of the hospice team members were of great assistance to both my father and my mother. This was an especially valuable asset due to the fact that both my sister and I were too far away to be of any practical help.

The hospice organization cared for him unit his peaceful and comfortable death in September, 2005. Hospice made an immediate difference in the lives of my parents and our entire family.

I chose hospice because I was impressed by the excellent care and treatment given to my father, which made a tremendous difference in my family's life. I was inspired to make that kind of difference in the lives of other patients, with a terminal illness, their families, and loved ones, too.

Thinking back over my hospice nursing career I am reminded of my most memorable experience. I recall a patient named Mary*who literally lived to watch "Dancing With the Stars," every week.

She expressed an interest in seeing the production "up close and personal."

Arrangements were made and tickets were obtained for the patient, her primary caregiver, and hospice nurse to attend a taping of the show. Her family said they had never seen her so excited.

With the patient's permission, prior to the taping, the hosts of the show had been told their special guest Mary*was a hospice patient. Before the show begin everyone in the production cast made an extra ordinary effort to meet with and welcome her.

Our patient was able to see the entire taping, and meet some of the performers. In spite of out to dinner with her on the way home!

The family was also very excited and pleased; they reported that their loved one told everyone with whom she came into contact about her adventure at "Dancing With the Stars;" she could not have been happier.

If I had not been before, at that time, I became fully aware that hospice is not only about death and dying. Sometimes it's about fun, and life, and helping terminally ill patients to make their last wishes come true.

A week after her 'adventure,' in a comfortable, relaxed state, and a mind filled with memories of a fulfilled dream, Mary* passed from this life to the next, with a peaceful death.

My name is Valerie Cook, RN, PCM. This is my Personal Testimony and I approve of it being published.

*Name changed to protect privacy and confidentiality

The Registered Nurse (RN) Case Manager

The Registered Nurse (RN) Case Manager Duties and Responsibilities include, but are not limited to, the following:

Upon assignment to a patient as Case Manager, the Registered Nurse (RN) develops and implements the patient Plan of Care (POC) and evaluates the nursing needs for each individual patient. Pain and symptom management and control are the RN Case Manager's primary focus.

The RN Case Manager works closely with the Medical Director and Attending physician to ensure that the patient's medical needs are being appropriately addressed and met, that pain and symptoms are being controlled, and that the patient is kept as free from pain, with needs met, and as comfortable as possible.

The RN Case Manager teaches patient and family about medications being prescribed, purpose for medications, and how and when to use them.

In addition, educates the patient and Primary Care Giver PCG) about the related hospice services which will be provided by the Interdisciplinary Group (IDG) Team, i.e., Medical Social Worker, Chaplain, Bereavement Coordinator, and the availability of a Volunteer, and also teaches safety measures so the patient's on-going safety and comfort is maintained at all times.

Finally, provides information about the terminal illness diagnosis, what to expect as the disease progresses, and how to respond in ways that will respect the patient wishes and will provide increased comfort to the patient.

SUMMARY

The RN Case Manager attends every Interdisciplinary Group (IDG) meeting coordinating patient care and, encourages every member of the Interdisciplinary Team to follow the patient Plan of Care (POC);

The RN Case Manager also provides the patient with as much independence as appropriate and possible, and to work with each team member, through the Interdisciplinary Group (IDG) meetings, providing a clear line of communication, ensuring that the patient's needs are met, that they remain free from pain, and comfortable.

A Testimony of an Active Practicing Registered Nurse (RN) Case Manager

Testimony of a Hospice Nurse by Trish Kulcsar

RN—Registered Nurse, CHPN—Certified Hospice and Palliative Nurse.

I write this testimony at the request of our Hospice Chaplain, Curtis Smith. He has patiently waited months for me to put together a testimony of my calling as a Hospice Nurse. Why it has taken me so long is difficult to say, but finally I am taking on this challenge to write in a few condensed sentences about my calling and one of my most memorable experiences in Hospice.

The call to become a Hospice Nurse came for me like a 'Mid-Life Crisis'—In my thirties, I decided to go back to school and have a complete career change. I was renting a room in a 3-Bedroom apartment in Orange County, California, when my roommate, Annette, who had become my closest friend, suggested I consider a nursing career. Annette was an LVN, disabled by Lupus and MS, raising her teenage daughter alone. She had great wisdom and compassion; I was very fortunate to have her friendship and encouragement. As an immigrant from Manchester, England, I felt I was well educated to a college level, and was on a successful career path of various jobs with Office Management and Sales & Marketing, with an Accounting background. The death of my first husband was tragic, he died so young at the age of 30 from colon cancer, but now the death of my second marriage was sufficient cause for me to question the path I was on. Was I on the path God wanted for me? My search for answers lead me back to College, and I graduated from Golden West with honors and a Registered Nurse License.

All through Nursing School the dramatic lessons carved into my heart made me determined not to work in the Hospital or a Skilled Nursing Facility, and yet I felt drawn to work with Geriatrics.

The ideal opportunity opened up for me with a Community Hospice and I knew this was the right path.

Now in my 50's and looking back over my twenty year nursing career, I see my previous job experiences have been an asset to help me handle the responsibilities of Hospice Case Management. For example, Sales & Marketing strategies have helped me during the difficult negotiations with patients and family members listening intently to an explanation of the palliative options of Hospice. I have a responsibility to know the 'Product' well, and so must have a thorough understanding of the rules and regulations governing the Medicare Hospice Benefit. Then you must 'Believe' in the 'Product' to present it well. I am convinced that the selling points of the Hospice philosophy are not only the focus on patient symptom management, but also that it has the unique medical model of identifying the physical, emotional and spiritual needs of the patient and caregivers as a unit, and is equipped with a Interdisciplinary Group of Professionals to collaborate and work together for the patient's, and caregiver's best outcome.

A common goal for patient and caregiver to express is, 'I desire a peaceful, comfortable death.' The patient, if able to express, would of course desire to be as pain-free as possible, and as alert as possible to have the most meaningful final moments with their loved ones. As a Hospice Nurse, we utilize our initiative and experience, becoming the eyes and ears of the physician, providing frequent written and verbal assessments.

Accurately updating the Hospice Medical Director and attending physician are crucial steps in striving to bring an optimal quality of living during the end of life. In order to fulfill this responsibility, the Hospice Nurse benefits from an increased knowledge of pathophysiology and the palliative treatment and medication options, in addition to an understanding of the dying process.

Finally, in sharing your knowledge and information, by compassionately teaching the patient and caregivers, the Hospice Nurse is often able to facilitate a more peaceful adjustment to the changes faced by both patient and loved ones, and by the surrounding caregivers.

In career reflection, perhaps the most memorable events in my Hospice experience have been tested by their dramatic outcomes; One recent case, was my patient, I will call her Martha; a successful career woman in her 50's. Single and never married, she had recently taken some time out of her busy schedule to care for her ailing mother. After her mother's death, Martha began to rapidly gain weight, and yet was losing her appetite and fatigued easily. Soon Martha learned that her increased stomach girth was something called ascites and that the recent years of excess alcohol consumption had borne heavy consequences. Martha was given a terminal diagnosis of liver cirrhosis; she declined aggressive treatments and did not want to consider a liver transplant. She moved to be near to her siblings and was admitted to a Skilled Nursing Facility for Hospice Care. After the Hospice admission process was complete I made an appointment to meet with Martha and her closest family member, her sister, I will call her Mary. Introductions went well, Martha was sitting up in her wheelchair, fully oriented, but her speech was slower due to hepatic encephalopathy. Her abdominal pain was moderately severe, self-measured at 6 out of 10. At first she was able to transfer independently from the bed to the wheelchair, and attend to her own bathroom needs.

She looked 10 months pregnant with ascites. I learned there were 4 siblings, and some strained relationships between some of them.

Martha wanted to connect with a real faith in God, but had not made the time to in the past, now she hesitated to, expressing she would let me know when she was ready to see the chaplain. Her sister Mary often spoke tearfully outside of the room and out of Martha's hearing, sharing stories of their family and of her own strong faith and about the many years of prayers given on her sister's behalf.

Within the first 3 weeks of General In patient Care, Martha's symptoms were aggressively addressed with daily Hospice nurse visits and with multiple changes in Doctors' orders she was reporting effective pain management of less than 2 out of 10, the majority of time. Mary and her brothers had various concerns about the patient condition changes, and ongoing education was helping them come to terms with their sister's palliative choices. But a sudden change of condition occurred that was unexpected by anyone.

Martha had been in the habit of wheeling herself down to a facility-smoking patio, at the front of the building. Martha had ran out of cigarettes that evening and decided to wheel herself to the store to buy more.

Sadly Martha was hit by a car and sustained multiple fractures, and lacerations. Miraculously, Martha remained alert and oriented and albeit bedbound from then on, yet she was able to talk with her sister Mary, and her other visitors. After the accident Mary prayed openly with her sister, and offered her spiritual support to Martha. Martha said she was ready to draw near to God, and gave her heart to Jesus, and after this she made many comments about feeling joy, and was often found smiling, saying. "I don't know why I am smiling, I just feel good." The Chaplain and Social Worker were actively involved in their emotional and spiritual support and Martha had a peaceful, comfortable death.

I was invited to attend her Memorial Service, and our Chaplain officiated. Mary eulogized her sister beautifully, and I felt honored to witness the miraculous healing that took place in Martha and her family.

I think having seen the majority of patients and caregivers meet their goal of a peaceful and comfortable death successfully, has been one of the main reasons for my long career with Hospice. There have, however, been a few cases that deeply grieved me, for one reason or another. Therefore in closing, I need to mention the enormous importance of personal physical, emotional and spiritual health. There is no doubt a great physical, emotional and spiritual demand upon the Hospice Nurse, and I cannot stress enough how immeasurable the blessings of frequent quality time off, good family, friends and church support are to the ongoing call.

Again, thanks to my colleague Curtis for giving me this moment of review, I trust it will be of encouragement to the few considering the challenges of this incredible Ministry of Hospice care.

My name is Trish Kulcsar, R.N. and I approve of this Personal Testimony being published.

*Names changed to protect confidentiality and privacy

Licensed Vocational Nurse aka Licensed practical nurse

From Wikipedia, the free encyclopedia

Licensed Practical Nurses (LPNs) are also known as *Licensed Vocational Nurses (LVNs)* in California and Texas and as *registered practical nurses (RPNs)* in Ontario, Canada. They are called *enrolled nurses (ENs)* in Australia and New Zealand and as *state enrolled nurses*

(SENs) in the United Kingdom.

United States

Main article: Nursing in the United States

Licensed Vocational Nurse (LVN) aka Licensed Practical Nurse (LPNs) work in a variety of health care settings, including Hospice Care. They are often found working under the supervision of physicians in clinics and hospitals, or in private home health care. In long term care facilities, they sometimes supervise nursing assistants and orderlies.

The United States Department of Labor's Bureau of Labor Statistics estimates that there are about 700,000 persons employed as licensed practical and licensed vocational nurses in the U.S.LVN and LPNs follow the rules of State Boards of Nursing. Requirements for taking boards usually include a clean criminal record and graduation from an approved accredited practical nursing program.

Education and training, depending on state requirements, may be vocational-based, hospital based, or college-based, and can vary from 9 month certificate programs to 3 years in time for certain specialties like pediatrics, surgery/anesthesia, or school nursing which usually require an associate degree in practical nursing.[1]

In Hospice Programs the LVN works directly under the supervision of a Registered Nurse (RN) sharing a patient case load. Generally, (with some exceptions) they perform the same Medical Services for patient care as the Registered Nurse (RN) Case Manager.

A Testimony of an Active Practicing Licensed Vocational Nurse (LVN)

My name is Samina Arenas. I am an active Hospice Licensed Vocational Nurse (LVN), a single mother, divorced for 9 years, responsible for two adult children.

After graduating with a two year Nursing Degree from Long Beach City College, Long Beach, California I started working in a Skilled Nursing Facility (SNF). I loved being with patients and was pleased to continue working for several years gaining valuable experience with on-the-job-training in a nursing career.

I became acquainted with a Registered Nurse (RN) Case Manager who was employed by a hospice agency. When she made her rounds visiting hospice patients residing in the health care facility where I worked we would engage in conversation

One day during our interaction she asked me if I had ever considered working as a nurse with patients in hospice care. I admitted that I did not know enough about hospice care to have ever considered it. She suggested I think about making a change from a Skilled Nursing position in a Health Care Facility (SNF) to becoming a hospice nurse. She also informed me that there was an opening for a Licensed Vocational Nurse at the hospice agency where she worked.

She told me that if I was interested, she would be pleased to refer me, and give me a favorable recommendation. I told her I would think about it, which I did. Eventually, I applied for the LVN position and was hired.

For the first few months I struggled, working in a new environment, undergoing new employee orientation, and having to drive to different geographical locations to perform nursing duties. The thought crossed my mind that maybe I had made a mistake. I am happy to say that I adjusted quickly, never looked back, and begin to enjoy a new challenge.

I absorbed myself in nursing work and started to believe that I was making a difference.

After being a hospice nurse now for 9 years, I have never regretted making the decision to change my career track. Hospice nursing has provided me opportunity for "hands on nursing" with terminally ill patients beyond expectation.

I have been privileged to interact with both patients and families. I am able to connect with the patient at their point of need whether it is medically, emotionally, or socially, in an unhurried way. Sometimes I struggle not to get too emotionally involved. I have had to learn how to set boundaries.

Working with terminally ill patients has softened my perspectives; my priorities have changed. I value every day that life has to offer. I have become a better parent; a better mother.

Reflecting on my years working as a hospice nurse, my memory keeps coming back to one of the most memorable experiences. I was scheduled to see a certain patient on Wednesday afternoon. A nagging premonition kept prompting me to see the patient Tuesday. I decided to follow my premonition. I arrived late in the afternoon and went directly to the patient's room.

Mrs. Johnson,* was a 91 year-old colon cancer patient, who had been receiving hospice care for 4 months. Entering her room I moved to her bedside. Her eyes were open and I thought I detected a slight smile of recognition. I observed her to be experiencing respiratory distress (difficulty in breathing). I adjusted the nose piece on her oxygen and increased the liters flowing into her nostrils. I put my arm under her shoulders and lifted her up, fluffed the pillow to make her more comfortable. As I gently eased her back down I heard a whisper voice say, "Thank you." Then a gasp, and silence; the breathing stopped, her body went limp. She died a peaceful death in my arms.

My name is Samina Arenas. This is my Personal Testimony and I approve of it being published.

*Name changed to protect privacy and confidentiality

Medical Social Worker (MSW)

Upon patient assignment Medical Social Workers make an assessment of patient needs and concerns, develop and establish a Plan of Care (POC), to include visit frequency.

The MSW's Assessment includes the psychosocial and spiritual needs for each patient and family member, and working with other team members to establish goals to meet those needs. They attend and participate in all Interdisciplinary Group (IDG) meetings.

The Medical Social Worker is a key member of the Interdisciplinary Group (IDG) and meets with the patient and family on a regular, on-going, as-needed basis. One of their main goals is to help the patient and family set goals, identify problematic areas, resolve differences, and cope more effectively, up to and including their suggestion to family members on how to say their final good-byes, as they move through the very difficult phases of anticipatory grief, death/dying, and the bereavement process.

During the assessment the Medical Social (MSW) will approach the subject death/dying, and pre-planning for funeral arrangements, selection of mortuary, etc. This is a very important and essential area of discussion which needs to be brought into focus with the patient and family.

With this recorded information in the patient's home chart it will be far less stressful and difficult—when the patient passes—for surviving family members to deal with the loss, and put into place the plans which have been decided upon.

The Medical Social Worker (MSW) also serves as a liaison referral guide for patient and family for referrals to outside of hospice support agencies, and to available local community services.

The Medical Social Worker (MSW) reports to the Patient Care Manager (PCM). They are directly responsible for regular, on-going, patient assessment to ensure that the patient's psychosocial needs are met and, that the patient is free from pain, and comfortable.

A Testimony of an Active Practicing Medical Social Worker

The name is Vivian Ro, MSW. I am a Hospice Social Worker for a private hospice agency in Southern California. I earned a Master's degree in Social Work (MSW) from the University of Southern California, (USC), Los Angeles, California. I completed undergraduate studies for a Bachelor's degree at the University of California, Los Angeles., California (UCLA).

Why did I choose Hospice?

When dealing with end-of-life issues, most people are not afraid of death but scared of the dying process. As a Hospice Social Worker, it allows me opportunity to connect the terminally ill and dying patient to community resources, to counsel their families, and offer, in an unhurried way, special time and needed attention.

Sometimes, interaction with the patient is brief, but I am honored to offer comfort and compassionate care to patients during their end-of-life journey. After working five years in the hospice industry, I am convinced this is a special, Providential calling for me to accept and be

The Hospice Social Worker assists the physician and other Interdisciplinary Group (IDG) team members to more fully understand the significant psychosocial and emotional dynamics related to the patient's health care issues.

Medical Social Workers participates in developing the patient Plan of Care (POC), their Treatment of pain and symptoms, prepare clinical and on-going progress notes, works with the family, refers and uses appropriate community resources, participates in discharge planning and In-service educational programs, as well as, acting as a consultant to other agency personnel.

As I reflect on my years in a hospice career, I recall the most memorable event that happened during the hospice experience.

I helped a patient named Cathy* fulfill her dream; to have a wedding ceremony before she died. When I first met Cathy, she was angry and in denial. She indicated to me that there was much unfinished business in her life, and that she was not ready to give up on living.

One goal was be a caregiver for her frail mother, instead of herself being cared for. She wanted to play with her grandchildren and help them with their school homework. Most importantly, Cynthia had not yet declared her love to her longtime partner Gary* by marrying him.

She also told me that, she was not yet ready, to say her final goodbye to her family. But, at the same time, she wanted to tell them just how much she loved them, but didn't know how. As a Medical Social Worker; I believed Cathy needed to tell her family how much she did love them. I also believed that her wedding ceremony would be a perfect way to help her to do that, starting with the most important person in her life.

My most memorable moment was seeing Cathy walk down the aisle. At that moment in time, she was not a patient with a terminal illness, but a beautiful bride who was living and fulfilling her dream.

This experience caused me to fully realize that, Hospice is not a prescription for death, in fact, it is about celebrating life. As a Hospice Medical Social Worker, I am honored, to be part of a hospice organization

My name is Vivian Ro, MSW. This is my Personal Testimony and I approve of it being published.

*Names changed to protect privacy and confidentiality

THE HOSPICE CHAPLAIN

The Hospice Chaplain, also known as Spiritual Care Coordinator, (SCC), and Chaplain, is an equally important and integral part of the hospice team, providing compassionate care to patients with a terminal illness diagnosis, and their families.

The Chaplain's distinct education, skill, experience, and sense of calling, uniquely characterize the spiritual care professional. When patients and families require professional spiritual counsel and care, they turn to the hospice chaplain.

Some of the Chaplain's spiritual support services available for the patient and the families are, but not limited to:

- Increased understanding, acceptance and coping through prayer, reading from sacred texts, sacraments or other services as requested by patient or family
- Assistance with patient and family issues of meaninglessness, loss of faith, failure, anger, despair, betrayal, fear/dread, guilt, grief, hopelessness, forgiveness, bereavement, and general questions about the meaning of life and death.
- Assistance with connecting or re-connecting the patient and family with a place of worship or religious affiliation, and assist with Arrangements for a clergy to visit patient's home
- Assistance with funeral or memorial service arrangements and Information about religious practices
- Officiate the patient's funeral memorial service, at the request of the family
- Provide bereavement counseling services for the family if requested for as long as needed
- They attend and participate in all Interdisciplinary Group (IDG) meetings.

THE MISSION OF THE HOSPICE CHAPLAIN

The profound mission of the Hospice Chaplain is succinctly encapsulated within two paragraphs in the forward to the *National Hospice and Palliative Care Organization* publication pamphlet under "Foundations of Spiritual Care in Hospice," page 2, which states, in part:

"The journey of dying provokes a heightened awareness of a person's morality, personal relationships and compelling spiritual issues. Dying is a profound rite of passage, sometimes mysterious and often filled with changes, suffering, distress and refining realizations for all involved. Concerned hospice professionals," ___ *especially* Chaplains ___ (author's comment) *"...are sojourners with patients in search for meaning, comfort, strength and hope. Practiced with reverence and compassion, in relationships of trust and mutuality, hospice care remains always essentially sacred and spiritual in nature.*

"Hospice brings to the end-of-life journey a wholistic philosophy and practice intended to help patients and families accomplish with dignity the out-comes of self-determined life closure, safe and comfortable dying and effective grieving... Spiritual care in hospice supports the exercise of each person's unique spirituality, with the hope that meaning and love may be found in the presence of suffering and death.

THE GOAL OF THE HOPSICE CHAPLAIN

To assist the patient to have spiritual peace of mind, with the best quality of life possible, in familiar surroundings, with family and friends present, to make the end-of-life experience as loving and comfortable as possible, for whatever length of life they may have, and to die a peaceful death with dignity.

A Testimony of an Active Hospice Chaplain

The Spiritual Counselor

The dry, hot wind of an early California summer brushed against my face causing beads of perspiration to collect under the rim of my glasses and spill down my cheeks; my glasses slowly moved down the bridge of my nose. Standing on the front porch of a white, wood-frame house, I pushed the glasses back into place, rang the doorbell a second time and waited. I thumbed through the paperwork describing the hospice patient I was scheduled to see.

I really didn't know what to expect. As a Spiritual Counselor, and member of the Hospice Team of professional caregivers, I had learned at a recent interdisciplinary team meeting that there was a need in this patient's life *beyond* the usual. Today, during the time in which I would be conducting a Spiritual Assessment, I was hoping the patient would be able to discuss his *special need* with me.

The door opened. I stared into eyes that were filled with emotional pain and a sense of helplessness in not knowing what to do about a soul mate that was dying. I was ushered into the home and led to a back bedroom. A window mounted air conditioner nosily labored to lower the temperature in the room where the patient lay in a hospital bed. The closed curtains cloaked the bedroom in a veil of semi-darkness. As my eyes quickly adjusted I extended my hand and introduced myself to the man I had come to see. He took my hand and expressed appreciation for my visit. His smile reinforced his words. A look of sadness soon replaced the smile. I became a witness to the pool of pain and grief surrounding the dying patient, and the woman who shared his life. Two months earlier Alfonso had been diagnosed with colon cancer and had been given three to six months to live. Without fully realizing it, like many other times along the journey of faith and pathway of life, I would become an implicit vessel carrying the love of God to this couple.

Alfonso, 87, and Yolanda,* 75, had met thirty years ago after both of their first long-term marriages had failed. They fell in love and started living together. Their intent was honorable; they had planned on getting married. They became busily involved in and intertwined with the lives of their children from both marriages.

The blended family consumed their time and energy. Their dilemma was heightened when they learned that their church would not recognize their divorce, nor would the church marry them. The intent to marry was placed on hold.

The months had slipped by; the years had turned into decades. They wanted to take care of this *unfinished* business and get married, even if they had to marry *outside* their church. Then the cancer diagnosis had been made. The disease had metastasized (spread) and exacerbated (increased in intensity) and again their marriage plan had been interfered with. Alfonso was no longer ambulatory. Incontinent of both bladder and bowel he was now bed bound. He could no longer leave the house even in a wheelchair. An application for a marriage license requires two signatures. How *could* they ever marry?

As their hospice Spiritual Counselor I felt a sense of responsibility in helping them to obtain their life-long dream. A talk with the Marriage Bureau of the Records Department of the County of Los Angeles revealed that there *was* a way. With a note from a medical doctor attesting to the disability of the groom, and his inability to come to the court house, and the physical presence of the bride at the court house, plus a Notary (which I happened to be at the time) as a witness would permit the couple to obtain a Confidential Marriage License, which would enable them to be legally married.

Transportation was arranged and a Confidential Marriage License was applied for and obtained by the bride. A date was set for the wedding. Family and friends were invited. With the bride standing beside the groom's bed the complete wedding ceremony took place including the groom kissing the bride. There was a sparkle in the eyes of both bride and groom when I, acting as the Spiritual Counselor officiary, pronounced them husband and wife, and introduced them as *Mr. and Mrs. Alfonso and Yolanda Ramirez.*

With a lump in my throat, and a chill racing down my spine, I realized I had performed a service for Mr. and Mrs. Ramirez that completed a chapter in their *"Book of Life;"* the *final* chapter. Alfonso Ramirez died three days later.

Names changed to protect Confidentiality and Privacy

When It's Time, Author, Dr. Curtis E. Smith, PUBLISHAMERICA Publishing Company, 2008, Baltimore, MD, 197 pages, quoted from pages 13-14, used with permission of author.

Another Testimony of an Active Practicing Hospice Chaplain

My name is Rev. Felix A. Colon. I have been a Minister since 1974. I received my education at the American College of Metaphysical Theology, Minneapolis, Minnesota with a Ph.D. degree in Biblical Studies, and at the California Graduate School of Theology, Rosemead, California with a Ph.D. (ABD) degree in Biblical Counseling.

My reason for choosing to work in the Hospice Field was to be able to provide spiritual support—from an ecumenical perspective—and on-going emotional support to terminally ill patients and their families, as they daily face the trauma and stress of dealing with the challenges associated with a loved one living with a life-threatening illness.

My responsibilities include, but are not limited to, providing translation (I am bi lingual) assessing spiritual needs, and providing counseling to patients, families and primary caregivers (PCG's) in a compassionate and timely manner. Additionally, to facilitate patient/clergy contact at the patient's request; developing and documenting a patient Plan of Care (POC), establishes visit frequency, and work closely with the Interdisciplinary Group (IDG) team members.

Reflecting on my hospice pastoral experience I specifically recall a memorable event. I was assigned a patient who was being re-admitted to hospice care, from another hospice agency provider. According to the family her initial hospice encounter had been very negative. The family recounted that she had been a difficult patient to please, with many complaints. They were skeptical about the loved one's new hospice care provider. Wanting to avoid whatever problems they had previously experienced, they were far more demanding than a typical family normally would be. The Interdisciplinary Group (IDG) team was quickly made aware of the prejudiced mind set of family members, and each worked hard to provide and monitor the quality of excellent care as is customary with hospice.

Over time, the patient experienced a rapid decline, and within days passed away. As their Chaplain the family asked me to officiate at the funeral memorial service. I agreed to do so.

The week following the memorial service, I received a very complimentary thank you note from the family, expressing grateful appreciation for the memorial service and for the excellent quality of care provided by the entire hospice professional team. A potentially negative situation was turned into an unbelievable and unexpected positive.

My name is Rev. Felix A. Colon, Ph.D. This is my Personal Testimony and I approve of it for publication

The Certified Home Health Aide (CHHA) aka Bath Aide; Home Health Aide

The Certified Home Health Aides aka Bath Aide, and Home Health Aide, is a very important member of the Hospice home health care team, who helps the patient to retain confidence and independent. Their daily/weekly routine duties include, but are not limited to the following:

Assist the patient with bathing; in-bed, shower or tub, and their toileting

To help with care of teeth, mouth, and oral hygiene

To aid with transfer of patient from bed to chair, chair to wheelchair, and in walking

Assist with grooming: hair, care of nails (not toenails), *and male patients* electric shaving

To aid in dressing the patient

If present at mealtime to help with serving nutrition and aiding patient feed self

To assist by providing patient overall hygiene

Assist patient with Durable Medical Equipment, safety and mobility, e.g. wheel chairs, Hoyer Lifts, Walkers, etc.

Remind patients to take medications on time (to be dispensed / given by family members)

Un-Authorized Activities

Give injections

Dispense/Give medications and/or suppositories

Change wound-care dressings

Make Medical judgments or offer Medical advice

As previously stated, the Certified Home Health Aides (CHHA) aka Bath Aide, is a very important member of the Hospice health care team in providing overall patient personal care, hygiene, and sanitation to ensure palliative and comfort care.

The CHHA works directly under the Supervision of the Registered Nurse (RN) Case Manager, who teaches them how to perform specific procedures to ensure ongoing, quality care.

A Testimony of an Active Practicing Certified Home Health Aide (CHHA)

My name is June Diacson. I am a Certified Home Health Aide (CHHA). I work with a hospice agency where my role is to provide personal care to terminally ill patients. I have become a career Certified Home Health Aide and have worked for my present employer for many years.

In order to become a Certified Home Health Aide I had to go to school, take and satisfactorily pass many examinations over the information I was being taught, and to eventually become certified in the state where I am employed.

I enjoy my career and I believe it to be a privilege to be able to work with patients who are dying. My goal is, to provide the best possible quality of personal care. Upon being assigned a patient I make a connection via the telephone and schedule an appointment to meet with both patient and family. When I meet the patient whom I will serve, and the family, I have learned to recognize just how important it is for me to present a friendly, and at the same time, professional demeanor with proper dress, and grooming. The first impression is very important for the patient and family ensuring that they will be comfortable with my presence.

My Role and responsibility, in patient care management, is to give baths, shampoos, and personal care to both female and male patients who have been diagnosed with a terminal illness.

After meeting with the patient I have to make a decision as to which type of personal care is most appropriate for them, i.e., a bath in bed, a tub bath, or a shower bath. My decision is based upon the physical condition of the patient as to how much physical exertion they can tolerate.

In providing patient personal care one of my biggest concerns is to make sure the patient is comfortable. Some patients have contracted arms and legs, or are in a fetal position, making it difficult for me to bathe them. I try to be very careful to make sure my interaction will not cause increased discomfort or pain.

I work with patients who are alert and oriented, as well as patients who are semi-comatose, or are in a comatose state, providing in-bed, tub, and shower baths to ensure patient continuing good hygiene.

If I provide personal care for a patient over an extended period of time, I discover a bond developing between us. In one way this is a positive aspect for me. In another, it becomes a negative; when I observe one of my patients begin to change, and start to transition from this life to the next. It touches my emotions to see them change from alert and oriented to become unresponsive, and then slide into a comatose condition.

As for me and my chosen profession, I have always known that in working with the terminally ill I could not provide good care and service if it didn't come from my heart. In giving good care I have always tried to follow the Golden rule of, *"Do unto others, as I would have others do unto you"(me)*.

I know that, by following this Biblical teaching, even when a patient become angry with me for no good reason, and lashes out at me, no matter how hard I try to please them, In my mind, it sometimes makes me feel like I have failed. Realistically, I know that I have made an honorable effort to reach my goal in providing the best possible quality of personal care service. It is then that I realize, and I know in my heart, I have not failed; I have succeeded.

In doing my work there are disappointing and sad times. Before I leave the home I usually say to a patient, "I'll see you next time." I have had some patients reply by saying, "I won't be here." Meaning that they would probably pass away prior to my next visit. Sadly, some had accurately predicted their own death; before my next visit, they did die.

As I look back over my hospice career, I recall the most momentous experience, and at the same time, the saddest and most difficult experience; that was when a patient I was bathing died in my arms.

At the end of the shift, my overall goal is to have given the best possible quality of care I am capable of giving, and continue to honor the bond which has been formed and established between the patient, family, and me as a gift to the patient and family; the gift of myself.

My name is June Diacson. This is my Personal Testimony and I approve of it for publication

The Primary Caregiver (PCG)

The Primary Caregiver (PCG) can either be paid, or volunteer. They are most often a family member. They provide ongoing care and support to the patient and family during the time the patient is under Hospice Care. They provide a direct communication link between the patient, family and the Hospice Interdisciplinary Team (IDG) of healthcare providers.

The term Primary care refers to the on-going, basic services provided for the patient's emotional and physical active daily living (ADL) needs. The overall concept and meaning and goal is for the Primary Caregiver (PCG) to be available, with their presence and compassionate caring as an active listener, for feel, touch and verbal stimuli communication.

Whether paid, or a volunteer family member, the Primary Caregiver (PCG) takes on a crucial role in providing care and support to the patient and family. If the Primary Caregiver is a 24 Hour, live-in Primary Caregiver, (PCG) they are often thought of as a surrogate part of the family. As the patient's disease progresses, and their needs change and become more intense, the Primary Caregiver (PCG) is turned to by family members for additional strength and support.

The Primary Caregiver (PCG) is a special type person, and a valuable part of the Hospice Healthcare Team, however, they are not authorized to make decisions for the patient and or family unless the patient has named the Primary Caregiver their Durable Power of Attorney representative.

In fact, in real time, the Primary Caregiver (PCG) position can be a very heavy and demanding role. It requires a time commitment for involvement of energy, compassion, unselfish love, and time spent with the patient and family members.

The Primary Caregiver's commitment enhances both the patient's and family's lives and, specifically, provides the patient with a sense of self-worth, respect and dignity.

The ultimate Primary Caregiver (PCG) goal, whether paid or a volunteer family member requires giving from a heart filled with love: an extraordinary gift; the gift of self.

A Testimony of an Active Practicing Primary Care Giver

My name is Betty Palao. I am a full time Primary Caregiver (PCG), working as a live-in 24 hour, 365 care giver in patient homes. I have worked in this career position for a number of years. As a spiritual person filled with a passion to care for others, I believe this is a work I have been divinely called to, i.e., assisting the elderly, infirm, and those with debilitating diseases in the final stages of their lives.

I have always been interested in observing how a patient's life can be so blessed, and at the same time, still not be spared from contracting a disease. How one can be so strong while daily facing the symptoms of a disease process—with their world slowly fading away—and still be able to maintain their faith in the Lord.

Being a Primary Care Giver (PCG) is not an easy job; one needs a lot of patience, determination, hard work and a keen, compassionate interest, in order to be successful in providing quality care for those patients with whom you serve. In my Primary Care Giver (PCG) role I have cared for different kinds of patients from the chronically ill to those with a terminal illness.

I remember one time I was caring for a 57 year-old female patient who, because of her strong faith in God, was able to bear very heavy pain brought on by her terminal illness. Even though, for the majority of time, the pain was being mildly controlled by prescribed pain medication, she continued to experience pain. It appeared as if there was never a day when she was totally pain free. She kept a Holy Bible at her bedside and it was refreshing to see her reading the Word of the Lord. This was a daily routine for her right up until the day of her passing. I was at her bed side when she passed; it appeared like she experienced a peaceful death, she died in her sleep.

I also remember caring for a terminally ill male patient in his seventies. Through shared conversation I learned that he had once been a faithful attendee at a local protestant church. For reasons he couldn't remember he had stopped going to church. In his own words he told me that he had 'not been inside a church in many years.' He had not only drifted away from the church, he had also turned away from God.

Over time, as we continued to discuss important matters, including faith, he asked me to pray for him that he could restore his relationship with God. I was pleased to be able to grant his request, and prayed with him, and for him. He later told me that, 'it was you who brought me back to the Lord.' While he gave me credit, in my mind and heart I refused to claim credit: I knew who *really* brought him back to the Lord. He seemed to have gained a burst of energy and strength and appeared stronger, not physically, but spiritually, which helped him a lot.

The privilege to share my compassionate care, concern, and my faith, is one of the most important dynamics of my Primary Care Giving (PCG) work. As a caregiver my role and responsibilities include providing comfort care, the basic need at this point in the patient's life, providing healthy and nutritious meals whenever and whatever is tolerated, hydration, and a clean, comfortable living environment.

As a caregiver I believe every patient should be treated in a concept of whole human needs, physically, emotionally, psychologically, and spiritually. In my opinion the caregiver should provide, not only a professional demeanor, but also demonstrate a friendly attitude, especially to those patients who live alone, have no one to talk to, and are isolated from frequent family contact.

Each patient presents unique experiences, and provides the opportunity, for me to meet my goal, of providing the best possible quality care for them, until they reach the destination to their end-of-life journey.

My name is Betty Palao. This is my Personal Testimony and I approve of it for publication

The Bereavement Coordinator aka Bereavement Counselor (BC)

The Bereavement Coordinator duties and responsibilities include, but are not limited to, the following:

To plan, maintain, and implement an effective Bereavement Program to meet, and satisfy, the needs of immediate family / loved ones, following the death of the Hospice patient. Hospice criteria provides for bereavement support to continue for thirteen months from date of death—or longer—depending on severity of survivor grief. They attend and participate in Interdisciplinary Group (IDG) meetings.

In a timely manner, following the death of a Hospice patient, coordinates and leads the Assessments and delivery, of bereavement services to family, caregivers, and Healthcare facility Personnel; and thereafter, for 13 months, remains in contact via telephone contact, mailings, and on-going evaluation needs.

The Bereavement Coordinator attends and participates in all Interdisciplinary Group (IDG) meetings, In-service Education Training, and any applicable committee meetings.

Provides one-on-one bereavement counseling, at the request of family members, and conducts regular Bereavement Support Group meetings for the bereaved spouses and family members.

Assists in planning and conducting meetings and services to meet Hospice personnel coping and support needs, i.e. In-services, Education, Memorial Services, and Training sessions.

Provides one-on-one bereavement counseling and support to Hospice personnel dealing with grief issues and provides referrals to community resources.

Networks with community resource organizations and maintains a referral source for referral services to callers from the community.

Conducts an Annual Evaluation of Bereavement Service Program for on-going development and fine-tuning enhancement.

Coordinates Quarterly and Annual Memorial Services to include Hospice Families survivors and Hospice personnel.

The Bereavement Coordinator (BC) works independently but welcomes and accepts in-put guidance from other members of the Interdisciplinary Group (IDG) and from members of the community.

Accepts and performs any other relevant duties which may be assigned.

A Testimony of an Active Practicing Bereavement Coordinator

My name is Rev. Gary Tucker, a licensed and ordained minister since 1994. A mid-life career change took me back to school and to ministry. In the role of minister I first served as a Minister of Pastoral Care in a community church, then as a Hospice Chaplain, which led to a Salaried position of Bereavement Coordinator, a position I have served in since 2006.

I am now, and have been, employed as a Bereavement Coordinator for the past four years with a major Home Health and Hospice Agency in Southern California.

My role includes, but is not limited to, meeting with patients and families when the patient is initially admitted to Hospice service.

First and foremost, pre-bereavement needs are evaluated and assessed. My responsibility is to provide one-on-one pre-bereavement counseling, at the request of family members, *prior* to the patient's death. And *after* the patient dies to interact with family members to assist in any possible way to provide bereavement counseling to assist in relieving anxiety and stress over the loss of a loved one in providing a sense of closure.

In a timely manner, following the death of a Hospice patient, it is also my responsibility to coordinate and lead the assessments and delivery, of bereavement services to family, caregivers, and thereafter, for 13 months, and to remain in contact via telephone, mailings, and on-going evaluation needs. In addition, to plan and conduct regular Bereavement Support Group meetings for the bereaved spouses, and family members.

Presently I conduct 5 Support Groups, at different times and locations throughout the county that the Hospice Agency I work for services. Two primary annual events planned and conducted by me include a Spring Celebration of Life, and a Fall Memorial Service for the bereaved, and their family members.

I thoroughly enjoy my career; I like meeting and working with patients and families from different cultures, ethnicities, faith and tradition backgrounds.

I am often asked to help clergy plan an appropriate worship service for those with early to mid-stage Dementia. This was a disease I knew least about prior to the start of my work with types of Dementia which have helped me to better understand the patients with whom I work.

It is truly a blessing working with the dedicated Interdisciplinary Group (IDG) team of hospice professionals during the last chapter of our patient's human journey, and then being able to help their families on their unwelcome and unfamiliar journey of life, after the death of a loved one.

My Name is Rev. Gary Tucker. This is my Personal Testimony and I approve of it for publication

Volunteer Coordinator (VC)

The Volunteer Coordinator organizes and oversees the overall Volunteer program to include, but not limited to:

To plan, maintain, and implement an effective Volunteer Training Program to meet the needs of patient and immediate family.

The Volunteer Training program curriculum would include an introduction to Hospice; the role of the Volunteer with patient and family; Care and Comfort skills; Communication skills; dynamics of death and dying; psychosocial dynamics associated with death and dying; safety; stress management; confidentiality, and patient rights.

Advertise for and solicit new Volunteers through word-of-mouth and In-service Training Sessions conducted at public high schools, hospitals, health-care facilities, and local community center.

Conduct Education Meetings for new Volunteers with specialized training enabling them to work to provide on-going companionship for patients and relief for families and the Primary Caregiver (PCG).

The Volunteer Coordinator attends and participates in all Interdisciplinary Group (IDG) meetings, Volunteer support group meetings, In-service Training for Volunteers, and Networks with community resource organizations and maintains a Hospice referral reference contact for referral by community organizations of callers from the community who want to become a Volunteer.

Conducts Annual Evaluation of the Volunteer Service Program for on-going development and fine-tuning enhancement.

Coordinates Quarterly and Annual Volunteer Appreciation Banquets / Dinners for Volunteer Recognition with Awards for meritorious Services, i.e., Volunteer with the most hours given to Volunteer Service; Volunteer of the Year; and Volunteer of the Month. Invitations are extended to include Hospice Family Survivors and Hospice personnel and families.

The Volunteer Coordinator works independently but welcomes and accepts in-put and guidance from other members of the Interdisciplinary Group (IDG), and from members of the community.

Accepts and performs other relevant duties that may be assigned.

A Testimony of an Active Practicing Volunteer Coordinator

My name is Judy Fassett; I am a Volunteer Coordinator for a large Hospice corporation located in Southern California.

I have worked with Hospice programs both in acute care medical facilities and in a free-standing hospice agency for the past five years

My duties and responsibilities include, but are not limited to, the recruitment, training, and retention of volunteers, and to maintain a quality, viable volunteer program within a Hospice organization.

I chose Hospice as a result of a personal experience with the imminent death of my own mother. I was deeply touched by the compassionate care giving Hospice gave to my mother. And after her passing I decided to become a Hospice volunteer. I worked as a Hospice volunteer for five years prior to becoming a paid professional Volunteer Coordinator.

I love my work. I choose not to think of my position as "work," rather, as a way of life. my ten years association with hospice has been rewarding with many moving, pleasant, and at the same time, sad experiences. I share an experience which I consider to be one of my most memorable.

I had the privilege of working with a patient who, over many weeks recorded her life review. For me, it was a moving and rewarding experience getting to know this person as a retired nurse, as a child, young lady, young war bride, and mature woman by being exposed to her life story. After her death it was particularly rewarding to present her family with her life in review. The families considered the recorded narration of her life review a gift to be able to hear in her own voice. Much later, one of her daughters told me, there were many stories their mothers and I had recorded that the family had never before heard.

My name is Judy Fassett. This is my Personal Testimony and I approve of it for publication

Hospice Volunteer

The Hospice Volunteer is a member of the local community who has a specific interest in wanting to help others. They work free of charge—without any remuneration whatsoever—including the cost of operating their vehicle, i.e. gasoline, mileage, insurance etc.

Often times the Volunteer is a surviving relative of a terminally ill family member who has been a hospice patient. Having observed the compassionate care and multiple benefits of a hospice program in action the volunteer is sometimes inspired to give back, through volunteer service, to the hospice community and thus becomes a Hospice Volunteer.

Prior to being approved as a Hospice Volunteer they undergo the same reference and background investigation checks that regular, paid employee would be subjected to. In fact, and in reality, they are considered to be an unpaid employee, without any employee benefits.

Volunteers are a very important and vital part of the Interdisciplinary Group (IDG). Their duties and responsibilities include, but are not limited to the following functions:

Volunteers provide on-going companionship for patients and relief for families and the Primary Caregiver (PCG).

The Volunteer provides many services such as offering patient care and comfort measures; providing emotional and psychosocial support; and offering a physical presence by just being there with the patient.

The trained Volunteer is available to assist the patient and family in multiple ways. They can remain with the patient while the Primary Caregiver (PCG) rests, or seeks a brief respite outside the home, away from the patient's presence; perform light housework and do other chores as is appropriate, and run errands or shop for the patient when requested.

The primary goal of the Volunteer—aside from offering un-selfish, compassionate care—is to make regularly scheduled supportive visits with the patient and family members, to be a friend and act as a companion.

The Volunteer reports to the Volunteer Coordinator and works directly under their supervision.

The Hospice Volunteer is one of the most valued services made available to patients and family.

Due to the close knit relationship and bonding a Volunteer has with the patient and family they are often considered to be a surrogate member of the family.

The Volunteer's motivation to serve, springs from a heart filled with care, compassion and love to offering the greatest of all gifts; the gift of self.

A Testimony of an Active Practicing Volunteer

My name is Ruth Gove. I am a Hospice Volunteer and Bereavement Telephone Caller to the bereaved. My responsibilities include making phone calls to those who have lost a loved one, assisting with bereavement support groups, and in addition I perform other assigned duties. I work for one of the largest hospice companies in the United States; I do volunteer work out of an office in Southern California. I have been a Hospice Volunteer for 17 years. I thoroughly enjoy doing the volunteer work.

I first became acquainted with hospice when my late husband was diagnosed with a terminal illness, and our family doctor recommended a Hospice program. I was very impressed with the professional quality of care, and kindness, both he and I received from the hospice staff.

Over the years I had performed volunteer work. I had received training through the church on visiting with, and by taking communion to the sick. After my husband passed away—while a hospice patient—I decided I needed to help others by becoming a hospice volunteer.

I have been blessed with many rewarding experiences. I share one experience that stands out in my mind. I had been assigned a patient named Bernie.* I visited with Bernie every Wednesday for three hours while the wife and daughter were out of the house. His wife and daughter told me that, "he doesn't know he is dying; please don't tell him." I told them I would honor their request. On my first visit Bernie said to me, "Your husband was on hospice, wasn't he?" I honestly replied, "Yes." He then asked, "How long?" I again gave him an honest answer, "One and a-half months." His reply was a simple, "O.K." I didn't say anything more to him remembering my promise to the family to not tell him 'he was dying.'

The next time I visited with Bernie he asked, "Did your husband die at home?" I replied, "Yes." On the next visit he asked, "Did he die peaceful?" Again, I simply said, "Yes."

I was scheduled to go on a 2 week vacation, and on the next visit I told Bernie 'I am going to be gone on vacation; I will see you when I return." Bernie said, "No. I will not be here then. Thanks for your kindness, help and friendship."

His wife and daughter had said 'he does not know he is dying.' My mind formed the words, "Oh, yes he does!" and in my heart I knew he did. During our time together we had developed a close bond of friendship; he felt safe, secure, and free to talk to me, rather than his family, about his approaching death. Bernie talked about his life; what made him happy, his favorite foods, books, and what a good life he had lived.

I told his nurse about our conversation and she said, "Oh, no! He's not near death." That Friday, Bernie died a peaceful death

My name is Ruth Gove. This is my Personal Testimony and I approve of it for publication.

*Name changed to protect confidentiality and privacy

Quality Assessment Performance Improvement Manager (Quality Manager)

The Quality Manager is responsible for managing and coordinating the clinical activities of the hospice program to assure compliance with acceptable standards of practice, applicable state and federal laws and regulations and hospice policies and procedures. The Quality Manager is also responsible for the overall implementation of current clinical standards and practices through the performance improvement process as well as through staff development and training. The Quality Manager is an integral member of the management team. The Quality Manager works collaboratively with hospice management to achieve the efficient and effective delivery of patient care resulting in positive patient outcomes which is achieved through the implementation of clinical standards and education.

In order to be successful in this position, an individual must understand and embrace the Hospice philosophy. The Quality Manager must be knowledgeable about Medicare Hospice benefits, eligibility, certification and acceptable professional standards and practices. It is also imperative that the Quality Manager is experienced in quality assessment and performance improvement methodologies, leading teams, data analysis, problem-solving and project management skills.

The Quality Manager coordinates with other clinical staff to identify opportunities for improvement relating to documentation and to identify effective methods to train staff in appropriate hospice documentation and techniques. This individual is responsible for conducting hospice staff education, coordinating new employee orientation and ensuring competency

The Quality Manager assures that hospice Quality Assessment Performance Improvement Program activities are effectively conducted, that opportunities for improvement are identified and works collaboratively to achieve performance improvement.

A Testimony of an Active Quality Compliance Manager

My name is Bonnie Stead. I have extensive experience in different aspects of Health Care Management. I have been actively employed in healthcare at various levels, from patient advocacy to health care management. These varied positions provided me the opportunity to gain experience in customer service, quality, health care compliance, instructional design and project management.

My preference always has been in the area of health care compliance and performance improvement. Therefore, three years ago I resigned an Information Technology and Project Management position to accept a Quality Management position with a major Hospice organization located in Southern California.

Before making the change, I evaluated my career track and realized that I desired a challenging and rewarding position, where I could utilize my experience and where people's lives could be impacted by what I do. Therefore, I applied for and accepted a position as a Quality Manager with a large Hospice Corporation.

My goal then, and is now, to use my skills to improve quality and assure compliance with acceptable standards of practice, applicable state and federal laws and regulations as well as hospice policies and procedures. I have now been employed in this position for three years and I thoroughly enjoy the challenges, the work environment, and my association with the people I work with.

Over the years I have had the opportunity to work for diverse organizations and manage personnel as well as interesting projects.

One of my most memorable and rewarding experiences was when I was working as a Compliance Manager at a major Medical Management Corporation. I was given the opportunity to lead this organization through a required survey for renewal of their limited Knox-Keene License. The corporation successfully passed the survey.

I must admit, though, nothing compares to working in the hospice field along with the compassionate individuals that care for the terminally ill at the end of their life's journey.

My name is Bonnie Stead. This is my personal testimony and I approve of it for publication.

CHAPTER 7

LEVELS OF CARE / TREATMENT

a. Routine Patient Care
b. Palliative Care
c. General In Patient Care
d. Crisis Care (Continuous Care)
e. Respite Care

There are five levels of care that are based on the patient's needs. The level of patient care is determined by the patient's need at the time of Admission. The various levels of care are listed here and briefly defined and described. This Hospice Guide Book presents an abbreviated overview of the different levels of care provided in Hospice. This Hospice Guide Book is not intended to be inclusive but serves to be an introduction to the various levels which can be provided under the Medicare / Medicaid Hospice Benefit Programs. Those levels of care are described and discussed as follows:

Routine Patient Care

Palliative Care

Continuous Care

General In-Patient Care

Respite Care

Routine Patient Care: This means the basic level of care under the Hospice Benefit Program.

At the time of Admission every component of the Interdisciplinary Group (IDG), as deemed appropriate, is assigned to that patient. The patient is notified that they will be contacted by each component to set an initial appointment for an assessment and or evaluation

The assigned Registered Nurse (RN) will schedule a time with the patient and family for an initial nursing assessment appointment. During the appointment time the RN will determine the modality of treatment to include frequency of visit, a Plan of Care (POC), appropriate medications, durable medical equipment (DME), and medical supplies needed, labs and diagnostic studies related to the terminal illness, as is appropriate, and any therapy services needed, such as occupational, speech, or physical.

The Plan of Care (POC) will specify the visit frequency for the RN Case Manager, usually 1-3 times per week, or more often, based on patient needs.

The Medical Director and the Attending Physician will closely monitor the patient's case, review their Medical Chart, and work closely with the RN Case Manager for medication orders, Medical Equipment, Medical Supplies, and other medical services as needed.

The Medical Social Worker will schedule an appointment for a patient evaluation assessment, to establish a Plan of Care (POC), and a visit frequency schedule for service, and to discuss and determine financial status needs, funeral and mortuary plans, psychosocial issues, and social service needs.

A Certified Home Health Aide (CHHA) aka Bath Aide will be assigned to the patient at which time a Plan of Care and visit frequency schedule will be established. The Bath Aide will usually visit 2-3 times per week (or oftener) based on the patient's need.

A major responsibility of hospice caregivers is to ensure that, at all times the patient is free from pain and comfortable. Therefore, each member of the Interdisciplinary Group (IDG) will assess the patient for pain at every visit.

If a member of the team observes the patient to be in pain, or is told by the patient that they are in pain, the team member will attempt to determine the location of the pain, and the intensity (pain level), so that the pain location and level of intensity can be reported to the RN Case Manager. The RN Case Manager will schedule an appointment to assess and address the pain level with necessary measures, to include giving the patient a pain medication treatment.

Counseling services will make an initial contact with the patient and Primary Care Giver in an attempt to schedule an appointment for a Spiritual Assess and Evaluation. Sometimes, when the Chaplain and the Bereavement Coordinator make the first contact with the patient, or family member, they make a decision as to the appropriateness and, as to whether either of these components are wanted at that particular time.

There will be times when; following the terminal diagnosis, there may be some hesitancy to discuss spirituality, death / dying, and pre-bereavement needs with a Bereavement Counselor Coordinator due to the trauma being experienced by both the patient and family. This is O.K.; it empowers the patient to know that they are still in control of their circumstances and, at the same time, gives them confidence to know that they can still make decisions on their own behalf.

Oftentimes, at a later date, the patient and / or family will decide they would like to welcome the Chaplain and the Bereavement Counselor into their home for pre-bereavement and spiritual discussion.

This is positive. It opens the door for additional support for the patient and family and, provides opportunity for, at least the patient, to make some decisions with regard to spirituality.

For as long as the patient remains on the hospice program they will receive regular assessments and evaluations, as is appropriate, and desired by the patient, from every component member of the Interdisciplinary Group (IDG), such as the Certified Home Health Aide (CHHA) for personal care, counseling, i.e., Pastoral, Spiritual, Bereavement, Dietary, and any other services deemed necessary.

Comfort Care, and patient freedom from pain, is the overall goal of Hospice Care. In hospice terminology this is called palliative care, aka comfort care, and will be defined and discussed in another section of this work, *A Hospice Guide Book*.

Under Routine Patient Care, previously discussed, *as with every other type of care provided*, the primary core value, focused goal, and purpose of Hospice Care, is to provide the patient with pain management, and controlled symptoms, medical care, emotional support, spiritual counseling for the dying patient, and emotional / spiritual support for the family

The basic difference between the various types of care is the dynamics involved with regard to medical personnel assignment, time frame involvement, location, and method of health care delivery, defined and discussed in the following identities.

Palliative Care

Palliative Care has previously been discussed however, it is rested her for clarity. Palliative Care focuses on making the end of life journey as comfortable and worthwhile for the Hospice patient. It provide a peace of mind that is reinforced by monitored medication and symptom control 24 hours a day, 7 days a week, with medical attention only a phone call away.

he Hospice Benefits Program delivers quality and compassionate care to patients who are facing a shortened life span due to a terminal illness diagnosis. The overall hospice and palliative care—by making available professional counseling support—enables the patient to deal with emotional and spiritual issues. The Hospice Benefits Program is customized to the patient's individual medical, psychosocial, social, emotional, and spiritual needs.

Palliative Care zeros in on reducing the level of pain, and the severity of symptoms of the terminal illness, rather than attempting to provide a cure. The goal is to make the patient as comfortable as possible, providing enhanced quality of life to include, medical emotional, psychosocial, psychological, and spiritual needs for whatever remaining time the patient has.

Hospice makes it possible for a patient, with a life-limiting illness, to face each day surrounded by loving, compassionate people who care, and live for whatever life remains, with loving attention, a sense of serenity, and die a peaceful death with dignity.

Continuous Care

When a patient develops out of control physical or emotional issue symptoms, which cannot be controlled with Routine Care, Continuous care becomes an option.

Continuous Care provides a more intense treatment model in the patient's home environment. A Continuous Care nurse, can be a Registered Nurse (RN)—but is usually a Licensed Vocational Nurse (LVN), in some states a Licensed Practical Nurse (LPN)—is scheduled to stay in the patient's home for a minimum of 8, and up to, 24 hours a day to administer pain medication treatments, symptom management control, and support until the pain and symptoms are under control

Example of symptoms which would require Continuous Care is: pain out of control; anxiety; nausea and vomiting; panic attacks; acute shortness of breath, and severe breakdown of the Primary Caregiver support.

Continuous Care is intended to support the patient through brief periods of crisis, i.e. with a level of care treatment option, exercised for short term periods. It is assessed and re-evaluated every 24 hours and, when the unrelieved pain, and uncontrolled symptoms have been brought under control the level of care is changed from Continuous Care back to Routine Care.

General In-Patient Care (GIP)

When a patient's pain level or symptoms becomes so severe that they cannot get adequate treatment at home General In-Patient Care becomes a viable option. If this option is exercised the patient is transferred from home to a General In-Patient facility. The basic difference between Continuous Care, aka Crisis Care, is the location of environment setting: the symptoms requiring In-Patient Care is the same as those requiring Continuous Care

With General In-Patient care nurses are available 24/7/365 to administer medications, provide treatments, and offer emotional support to ensure patient on-going comfort.

Three types of facilities provide General In-Patient services. They are:

1. **A Hospice House:** This is a free-standing facility usually owned and operated by a Hospice agency company and is staffed 24/7 with trained hospice staff members. Hospice Houses are a unique setting and are limited in number throughout the United States. Subsequently, due to the limited number of existing

   Hospice House facilities availability may not be an option at the time of need.

2. **Health Care Facility; Long Term Care Facility:** A hospice agency may lease, or sign a contract with a Skilled Nursing Facility (SNF) or Nursing Home usually consisting of a 4-6 bed unit / wing in, to provide care for General In-Patient status patients

3. **An Acute Care Hospital:** As with the Long Term Health Care facility a Hospice agency may lease a unit in the hospital to provide hospice General In-patient care with Hospice trained staff to provide around the clock In-patient care. Or the Hospice agency company may also have a contract with a hospital which would allow the hospital to provide 24/7 around the clock care for General In-patient service. In either case the Hospice agency company would provide supplemental care, per the Plan of Care (POC), with the trained Interdisciplinary Group (IDG) team.

Respite Care

Respite Care is designed more for the family and Primary Caregiver (PCG) than the patient. This level of care is used when the family is having a difficult time coping and may be overwhelmed with caregiver issues.

Caregiving can be very demanding and stressful causing the family and Primary Caregiver (PCG) to become stressed out, and overwhelmed with caregiver issues.

The purpose of the Respite Care is to provide a temporary relief (a time-away) from the duties of caring for the patient 24/7/365.

Respite Care provides a brief break, or respite to the patient's family and Primary Caregiver by admitting the patient to a health care facility.

In order to allow the family and Primary Caregiver a break (a time-out), from the duties of caring for the patient the Medicare Hospice Benefits will pay for a period of 5days of Respite Care in a health care facility

The Interdisciplinary Group (IDG) Team continues to follow the patient Plan of Care (POC) and provide the same needed and necessary services which would be provided in the home care setting.

NOTE: The patient can be admitted to hospice at any level of service, (except respite). The patient's condition determines the appropriate level of service, and depending on patient need, the level of service can be adjusted and changed back and forth at any time.

Patient Discharge from Hospice:

The subject of patient discharge from hospice needs to be discussed. There are a number of reasons a patient can be discharged:

Voluntary Discharge: A patient my voluntarily elect to discontinue Hospice care at any time, for any reason. Such as:

Revocation: If a patient refuses to cooperate and becomes totally non-compliant with the Hospice Benefit required regulations they are subject to and are usually requested to revoke hospice services.

Aggressive Treatment: When a Hospice patient decides they want to pursue aggressive medical treatment for possible cure they will then voluntarily revoke for that reason.

Transfer to another Hospice: Sometimes a patient becomes dis-satisfied with certain Hospice agencies and elects to transfer to another agency.

Moving out of Hospice Service Area: Occasionally a patient will re-locate to another city, county, or state and are geographically outside their current hospice agency provider service area. Subsequently, they are discharged for that reason.

Discharge for Extended Prognosis: Discharge for Extended Prognosis is, when a patient does not continue to decline by reason of weight loss, decreased appetite, decreased energy and strength, reduced cognition, and many other symptoms, during the initial 3 month Certification period, their case will be collaborated on for consensus by the Interdisciplinary Group (IDG) as to whether they remain hospice appropriate. If a patient does not continue to sufficiently decline, to meet the Hospice Benefit mandated guideline criteria, they will not be re-certified. They are then discharged for reason of Extended Prognosis. When the patient's condition again starts to decline and change they can immediately be re-admitted to Hospice.

Discharge / Revocation: When a patient becomes totally non-compliant with Hospice Benefit required regulations they are subject to revocation. A Hospice agency is not permitted to arbitrarily Revoke a patient; the patient must request to be Revoked.

Discharge for Aggressive Treatment: When a hospice patient decides they want to pursue aggressive medical treatment for possible cure then they will voluntarily revoke for that reason.

Death: When a patient dies, there is an automatic discharge by reason of death, their name is removed from the Hospice census roster.

CHAPTER 8

_____

RESIDENCES AVAILABLE

a. **Private Home With a Primary Care Giver**
b. **Board and Care**
c. **Assisted Living**
d. **Hospice House**
e. **SNF—Skilled Nursing Facility**
f. **LTCF—Long Term Care Facilities:**
   Primarily Provided for Alzheimer / Dementia Patients

There are 6 different kinds of residences used in providing Hospice Care. They are listed at the start of this chapter. These various kinds of residences will be briefly identified, defined, and described as follow:

Private Home with a Primary Caregiver:

Most Hospice patients are cared for in a home setting usually with a family member providing Primary care. Each patient is unique and the Plan of Care (POC) by the Primary Caregiver (PCG) is customized and tailored to that particular patient's needs.

Home Care services fall into two categories described as: Home Care Services, and Non-Medical Home Care. However, the term Home Care is often used synonymously. In fact, when the term Home Care is used, it implies services from the Non-Medical to Skilled Care. It is the intent and purpose of both to enable the patient to live independently and safely in the security of their home environment.

83

Home Care Services *per se*, is in fact, Medical Home Care. It involves skilled nursing care within the home that can only be performed by *licensed* personnel.

Non-Medical Home Care is more of a general nature. These services usually involve assisting the patient with the activities of daily living (ADL's) such as: dressing; grooming; personal care, meal preparation; light housework, and providing transportation, etc.

Remaining in the home provides a safe and secure environment for the patient and offers opportunity for the patient to be surrounded by caring, compassionate family members, and friends, in a familiar setting.

The hospice Interdisciplinary Group (IDG), a team of professionals, support the patient and the Primary Caregiver PCG), providing Hospice care services.

The Hospice goal is to make the patient as comfortable as possible and, at the same time, address on-going quality of life needs, i.e., medical, physical, psychological, psychosocial, pre-bereavement, and spiritual, to provide the best possible quality for whatever life remains.

Board and Care Residence

The primary purpose of a Board and Care facility is to provide home base care services to dependent care groups such as elderly, developmentally disabled, and the mentally challenged.

Board and Health Care facilities are not licensed to provide skilled nursing services (unless there is a credentialed Registered Nurse (RN) or Licensed Vocational Nurse (LVN)working in the home.

The Board and Care Health Care facility is permitted to assist the patient with their activities of daily living (ADL's) such as bathing, dressing, eating, personal care, hygiene, toileting, urinary and bowel incontinency care.

The Board and Care facility located in a residential community is small enough to be family oriented and large enough to be effective in providing patient needed and necessary care. The small, residential Board and Care facility is usually licensed 2 to 6 residents and provides a safe, comfortable, dignified environment for those who need assistance with their activities of daily living (ADL's) throughout the day and night.

Board and Care in a residential community is cost effective. The average monthly cost for care varies, however, on average the cost is about half for residential care in comparison to nursing home care.

For the individual who is compromised either physically, or mentally, and not able to live independently, the Board and Care residential setting can provide a safe, secure, dignified, family oriented, ideal environment

In a Board and Care facility the Hospice Interdisciplinary Group (IDG) team of professionals provide the same services to the hospice patient that they would normally receive in their own home; only the environment changes.

Assisted Living Health Care Facility

Assisted Living facilities are not retirement centers *per se*. They are specifically designed for the purpose of caring for the elderly who can no longer live independently on their own. The sizes of the Assisted Living facilities vary to accommodate from 20 to 200 resident patients.

The resident care consists of assistance with patient bathing, toileting, incontinence of bladder and bowel, dietary requirement, and supervision of medications.

Assisted Living facilities are not permitted to offer or administer what is considered to be medical services such as injections, colostomy care, or wound care. These are usually offered by community home health agencies that are contracted with the Assisted Living facility to provide these services consistent with frequency of need.

This technique for overall resident supplemental, multi-tiered care giving, provided in a friendly environment _ with professional care givers _ has proved to be very effective in helping the elderly hospice patient to live comfortably and to maintain a level of independence with dignity.

A Hospice House

A Hospice House is a private facility owned and operated by a hospice agency. These facilities are staffed by trained professional hospice staff and vary in size from 20+ to 200+ patient capacity.

They are usually located in a quiet, residential community easily accessible to people throughout the county.

The average terminally ill hospice patient wants to be cared for in the privacy, comfort and familiarity of their own home. Assisted by family as care givers and visiting hospice Interdisciplinary (IDG) team members many people are able to do so. However, for some staying at home isn't possible. Because they cannot be cared for in their own home some choose to become a resident in a Hospice House where people can feel comfortable loving in a home-like environment.

Those patients who can no longer be cared for and live in their own home would, under ordinary circumstance, have received care in hospitals or nursing homes. However, the Hospice House concept gives them an alternative residence while in a Hospice Program. An environment where they can be surrounded by family and, at the same time, receive excellent, comprehensive, and cost effective care focused on the individual's needs

The overall concept of a Hospice House program is to provide the patient with a trained team of professionals, who join in a common effort, with the patient and the families, to control pain, manage symptoms, and create a friendly, environment and an atmosphere of emotional, social, spiritual, comfort and support.

Basically, the services provided in a Hospice House are the same as those provided in a home care setting.

The patient is surrounded by an Interdisciplinary Group (IDG) Team of professionals consisting of a Medical Director, Hospice House Manager, Patient Care Coordinator, Registered Nurses (RN's), Licensed Vocational Nurses (LVN's), Nursing Assistants, Social Workers, a Chaplain, and Volunteer, all who jointly care for the patient.

When a Hospice patient or family decide to use a Hospice House facility *there may not be* a Hospice House located in their particular vicinity. Therefore, what could be perceived as a disadvantage for Hospice Houses facilities is, they are very limited in number, location and availability. Subsequently, the patient and family's intent to place the patient in a Hospice House may not be an option due to lack of availability in their geographical area.

Skilled Nursing Facilities aka Nursing Homes

Nursing Home Care typically involves providing and managing complex and / or potentially serious medical issues to include, but not limited to, coma care, tube feeding, infections, wound care, and IV Therapy.

Both short term and long term care is provided for those with serious medical problems and disabilities and others who are bedbound, wheelchair bound, totally non-ambulatory and are need dependent for all Activities of Daily Living (ADL's), with maximum assist.

Typically, Nursing Home Care is provided for those patients who have a serious disability to the extent that the services they need cannot be found through residential care, i.e., Board and Cares facilities, or home care.

For the hospice patient who sustains a hip fracture and will need rehabilitation after discharge from the hospital Nursing Homes provide rehabilitation services after a hospitalization for injury or illness that are typically used on a short-term basis.

Most of the costs in whole or in part will be covered by Medicare with the requirement that there is hospitalization for 3 days prior to a discharge to a Nursing Home.

The implementation of the Prospective Payment System limits payment to a Nursing Home and allows them to determine who they admit. This provision is designed for those patients who are on a limited budget and cannot afford to pay for Home Care costs

For residential care the patient may have to be placed in a Nursing Home with costs paid by the state in which the patient resides under Medicaid long term care program, designed especially for those patients with no financial resources who are financially destitute.

Many people erroneously believe that Medicare pays all costs for Nursing Home stays. Medicare only pays for the stay while the patient is receiving actual medical services for up to 100 days, provided that the hospitalization requirement has been met.

Medicare will only continue to pay for skilled care as long as the patient is responding to that care. Once the patient has reached a plateau where the Medical Doctor (MD) feels that the patient will not benefit by any further care, Medicare will stop making payment. Also, no matter what the needs, Medicare will only pay 100% for the first 20 days. From day 21-100, the patient will pay a proportionate amount per day, and the full cost after 100 days. Medicare will cover the total costs if the individual patient qualifies both financially, and physically, for long-term care.

A Brief Overview Explanation for Medicare and Medicaid Hospice Benefits are listed:

Medicare: When a patient is terminally ill and receiving Social Security benefits Hospice Care is covered under Part A for which there is no charge to the beneficiary. All other Medicare services continue under Parts A & B.

Medicaid: As of 2006, (latest figures available at this writing), 45 states plus the District of Columbia offer low-income patients Hospice Care as a cost covered Medicaid benefit. In general the Medicaid benefits are equal to the Medicare benefits.

Charity Care: Under Medicare law, no person may be refused Hospice Care due to inability to pay. Each hospice agency employs a financial specialist to answer patient questions about eligibility for receiving financial assistance.

Tricare: Tricare is the Healthcare Benefit program for active and retired Military personnel. Hospice Care is a fully funded benefit under Tricare. NOTE: Only Medicare certified hospice agencies can provide hospice benefits to Military personnel through Tricare.

Private Insurance: The majority of insurance plans issued by employers and managed care plans offer Hospice Benefits. With variation their coverage parallels the Medicare benefits.

Private Pay: When the patient does not have insurance or the insurance coverage is insufficient, the patient and family can discuss with the healthcare providers private pay plans.

For clarification, before taking any action, Medicare and Medicaid Hospice Benefits *should always* be discussed with knowledgeable health care providers.

For Hospice patients, Medicare, Medicaid, and patient cost benefit services can be fully explored, explained, and discussed with the Hospice Medical Social Worker.

NOTE*:* This information is provided for educational use and enlightenment only; *it is not intended* to be used for Medical Advice, regarding Medicare or Medicaid eligibility requirements and, or Medicare payment.

The information presented here was *current* and *valid* and in force at the time of writing and publication of this Hospice Guide Book. **Time, and over budget cost conditions, often reduces and limit Medicare / Medicaid payments and reimbursements.**

It is important for the individual(s) who may consider using Hospice Care to request all current and pertinent Rules and Regulations from the Hospice agency provider of choice.

Additionally, Medicare / Medicaid benefit eligibility, regulations, requirements, and Federal laws *may change* with the implementation of the Health Care Reform Bill passed in 2010.

It is important to check with the Hospice Medical Social Worker for the most current cost provisions for military, state Medicaid, and federal Medicare Hospice Benefit programs.

Long-Term Care Facilities (LTCF)—Primary Care for Alzheimer/Dementia Patients

Long-term care is when a patient requires someone else to assist them with physical or emotional needs over an extended time period.

This help and or assistance may be required for the patient's activities of daily living (ADL's). Not unlike other health care facilities these services are listed in brevity including, but would not be limited to:

Administering Medication	Feeding
Attending to Medical Needs	Grooming
Assisting with use of Medical Equipment	Helping with incontinence
Bathing	Meeting doctor appointments
Counseling	Managing pain
Dressing	Providing transportation
Doing laundry	Providing comfort and assurance

Patients who are receiving Medicare benefits and who have limited income and/or resources may be eligible for assistance in paying for their room-and-board out of pocket medical expense from a state operated Medicaid program.

Referred to as "dual eligible," there are various benefits available to low-income patients who are entitled to Medicare and would be eligible for some type of Medicaid benefit. When a patient qualifies for both Medicare and Medicaid, the coverage is referred to as, "Medi-Medi" however, in order to be eligible for Medicaid the patient has to have less than $2,000. in assets, and *income insufficient* to pay for the cost of care. A patient must be financially destitute in order to qualify for Medicaid.

The Hospice Medical Social Worker can assist the patient and family in assessing both Medicare and Medicaid benefit eligibility.

CHAPTER 9

PAIN AND PAIN MANAGEMENT

Definition: Since pain is a feeling; a symptom that cannot be accurately and subjectively assessed, the accepted criteria is then defined by the patient. Pain is very personal and unique to the patient's that is experiencing it. That is, *"pain is whatever the patient experiencing it says it is*. It is what it is.

Pain can either be physical or emotional; or simultaneously, a combination of both.

From Wikipedia, the free encyclopedia, we can learn that: "Pain is when any part of the body is hurt or sick. Nerves in that part (of the body) sends messages to the brain. The message that the nerve sends to the brain is called nociception. Those messages tell the brain that the body is being damaged. Pain is not just the message the nerve sends to the brain. It is the bad emotion *felt* because of that damage."

Kinds of Pain: There are two kinds. They are: *Acute* and *Chronic*

> *Acute* pain is short lived; only happens for a short time

> *Chronic* can last a long time; this type pain is of long duration

Types of Pain: There are four different types. Pain can be caused by different sources.

For example:

Cutaneous pain is caused by injury to the skin.

Visceral pain is caused by damage to organs inside the body

Somatic pain is caused by muscle, bone or joint pain

Neuropathic pain: there is no identified underlying cause.

This type pain occurs simply because the nerves are not working appropriately.

Recognizing Pain

It is a Hospice requirement for team professionals to assess the Hospice patient for pain at every visit with the patient. There are two methods for assessment.

The Verbal Patient:

When the patient is verbal they can be asked if they are in pain; or if they hurt anywhere.

If the answer is "Yes," and the patient affirmatively responds to the question of pain, the next step is to determine the location of their pain.

Locating the Patient's Pain:

The clinician asks the patient to place their hand over that area where they feel the pain, or, to point to the place where they feel the pain.

Determining the Level of Pain:

When the patient identifies the location of their pain the next determination is to assess the pain level. This is accomplished with the verbal patient by using a 0 to 10 Scale, i.e. by asking the patient:

"On a scale from 1 to 10, 10 being the highest, tell me how much pain you are having."

The Non-Verbal Patient:

When the patient is non-verbal, they need to be assessed for pain by observation. Some common signs and symptoms used to recognize pain in the *non-verbal* patient are:

anxiety	depression	moaning
agitation	frowning	pale
combativeness	grimacing	perspiring / sweating
clinched fist	groaning	restlessness
constantly shifting in bed	gritting of teeth	writhing

Treatment of Pain:

When a patient claims pain, and indicates the location, the best treatment is to stop the damage being cause by the pain identifying the source of the pain.

Once or cause has been identified the appropriate pain medication treatment can begin. There are many difference kinds of pain medicines available. The treatment model to be used depends entirely on the kind of pain being experienced by the patient. The determination chosen model will be left to the educated medical knowledge of both the RN Case Manager, and the

Attending Physician aka Primary Care Physician

In providing Hospice care a common pain medication diagnosed for moderate to severe pain is called Morphine Sulfate; for oncologist doctors and hospice doctor Medical Directors it is considered the "gold standard," medication for moderate to severe pain.

Pain medication addiction:

There is a concern by some patients and their care givers that consistent dosages of a pain medication can cause the patient to become addicted. There is always an unpredictable risk, for unexpected side-effects, from some pain medications. However, the risk of addiction is very low when prescribed medications are used with appropriate medical supervision.

Some people who have previously been addicted, to either prescription or street drugs in the past, have an increased risk of becoming addicted to prescribed pain medication.

When medications are dispensed by responsible party family members—and taken by patients under reliable medical supervision exactly as prescribed—the risk of addiction is greatly reduced.

CHAPTER 10

ADDRESSING ("911") EMERGENCY TREATMENT

a. **DNR—<u>Do Not</u> Resuscitate**
b. **Full Code—<u>Do</u> Resuscitate**

DNR—Do Not Resuscitate:

Resuscitation is a method of restoration of life or consciousness of an individual apparently dead or dying. According to Jonas: Mosby's Dictionary of Complementary and Alternative Medicine, "Restoration of vital signs for a person in cardiac or respiratory failure. Cardiac massage and artificial respiration techniques are employed, and fluid and acid-base imbalances are corrected."*

*Jonas: Mosby's Dictionary of Complementary and Alternative Medicine © 2005 Elsevier

When a patient is admitted to Hospice care they are requested to sign a statement choosing Hospice care. Subsequently, they are asked to sign a **Do Not Resuscitate (DNR)** agreement form.

Since the Hospice certification is based on proximity to death, i.e., live expectancy of 6 months or less, the objective for signing both agreement forms is to eliminate the need for excessive 911 calls and frequent hospitalizations.

It is not a mandatory requirement at the time of admission for a patient to sign a Do Not Resuscitate (DNR) form, and the subject is approached by hospice personnel with care and sensitivity.

If the patient refuses to sign the Do Not Resuscitate (DNR) agreement form at the time of admission it doesn't prevent the patient from being admitted to hospice care.

The Hospice personnel explaining Hospice Benefits should make it very clear to the patient and family that signing a statement choosing hospice care means giving up the choice for aggressive treatments and accepting the fact that death is imminent.

DO Resuscitate aka Full Code

In cases where the patients does not sign a Do Not Resuscitate (DNR) agreement document, they will be classified as a "Full Code," patient, which means that, in the event of a cardiac arrest (heart stoppage), or heart attack, they will be resuscitated usually by Para Medics after a 911 call.

The 911 call sets in motion a "Code 3" call out of emergency vehicles i.e., the local police, the fire department, and the Para Medics rolling to the scene with lights and sirens sounding, with all anticipated needed and necessary emergency equipment to provide emergency services,

When a 911 call is made for a patient emergency the Para Medics are required by law to use every possible measure to rusticate and transfer the patient to the closest hospital emergency room.

Normally, under Hospice Benefits care, only the 911 emergency services provided to the patient would be a medical need directly related to the Terminal Diagnosis. That is, emergency 911 facilitation and transfer of the Hospice patient to an emergency hospital room would be the responsibility of the patient and family if the medical need is not directly related to the Terminal Illness Diagnosis.

For Example: If a patient diagnosed with end-stage cancer elected Hospice care and, at the same time, they also had been diagnosed with a heart condition, the patient may refuse to sign a Do Not Resuscitate (DNR) agreement document. In case of a heart attack, the Hospice Benefits coverage would pay for the patient's use of 911 emergency services; this would be considered a covered patient benefit condition for comfort care.

As soon as the patient's heart condition was again stabilized they would be discharged from the hospital and transferred back to their home.

In cases where a patient elects Hospice care, and there is not an accompanying disease necessitating emergency care, and the patient refuses to sign a Do Not Resuscitate (DNR) Form document, the Hospice agency personnel will work with the patient, and family, to provide time for them to adjust to the terminal diagnosis, and counsel with them to determine the best time to have the patient sign a Do Not Resuscitate (DNR) document.

It is important for the Hospice personnel admitting a patient to Hospice Benefit care to make it very clear to the patient that they have the choice to discontinue and opt out of Hospice Care at any time and return to a curative care status for aggressive treatment.

CHAPTER 11

THE END OF LIFE'S JOURNEY

a. **Signs and Symptoms of Death and Dying**
b. **Stages of Grieving**

Q. What are the signs of approaching death?
In: Death and Dying
Hospice & End Stage Help
Hospice and Caregiver Support Information on End of Life Stages
www.tlchomehospice.com/hospice.html

A:
The dying process occurs in two stages: the pre-active stage of dying and the active stage. The pre active stage may last about two weeks, while the active stage of dying lasts about three days.

Symptoms of the pre-active stage include restlessness, agitation, social withdrawal, increased sleep, decreased appetite and drinking, pausing in the breathing, speaking about dead relatives or friends, swelling of the hands or legs, or requests to settle financial or family affairs.

Symptoms of the active stage of dying may include coma, hallucinations, longer pauses in the breathing, very rapid breathing, lung congestion, inability to drink, urinary or bowel incontinence, dark color of the urine, a dramatic drop in blood pressure, very cold hands and feet, numbness in the legs or feet, a bluish or purple coloring to the person's arms, hands, legs, and feet.

Answer

Because this is such a sensitive question and one we all think of from time to time (some fearing it, others able to cope with it) when we know it can happen at any age and not just to the elderly a more informative explanation is needed. I have been through this process many times, recently my own mother and the following information is excellent.

The following is from a Hospice and the copyright allows the original copy to copies with the stipulation that no alterations are made and that the name of the Hospice is shown:

Preparing for Approaching Death

When a person enters the final stage of the dying process, two different dynamics are at work which are closely interrelated and interdependent. On the physical plane, the body begins the final process of shutting down, which will end when all the physical systems cease to function. Usually this is an orderly and undramatic progressive series of physical changes which are not medical emergencies requiring invasive interventions. These physical changes are a normal, natural way in which the body prepares itself to stop, and the most appropriate kinds of responses are comfort enhancing measures.

The other dynamic of the dying process at work is on the emotional-spiritual-mental plane, and is a different kind of process. The spirit of the dying person begins the final process of release from the body, its immediate environment, and all attachments. This release also tends to follow its own priorities, which may include the resolution of whatever is unfinished of a practical nature and reception of permission to "let go" from family members. These events are the normal, natural way in which the spirit prepares to move from this existence into the next dimension of life.

The most appropriate kinds of responses to the emotional-spiritual-mental changes are those which support and encourage this release and transition.

When a person's body is ready and wanting to stop, but the person is still unresolved or unreconciled over some important issue or with some significant relationship, he or she may tend to linger in order to finish whatever needs finishing even though he or she may be uncomfortable or debilitated. On the other hand, when a person is emotionally-spiritually-mentally resolved and ready for this release, but his or her body has not completed its final physical shut down, the person will continue to live until that shut down process ceases.

The experience we call death occurs when the body completes its natural process of shutting down, and when the spirit completes its natural process of reconciling and finishing. These two processes need to happen in a way appropriate and unique to the values, beliefs, and lifestyle of the dying person.

Therefore, as you seek to prepare yourself as this event approaches, the members of your Hospice care team want you to know what to expect and how to respond in ways that will help your loved one accomplish this transition with support, understanding, and ease. This is the great gift of love you have to offer your loved one as this moment approaches.

The emotional-spiritual-mental and physical signs and symptoms of impending death which follow are offered to help you understand the natural kinds of things which may happen and how you can respond appropriately. Not all these signs and symptoms will occur with every person, nor will they occur in this particular sequence. Each person is unique and needs to do things in his or her own way. This is not the time to try to change your loved one, but the time to give full acceptance, support, and comfort.

The following signs and symptoms described are indicative of how the body prepares itself for the final stage of life.

Coolness

The person's hands and arms, feet and then legs may be increasingly cool to the touch, and at the same time the color of the skin may change. This is a normal indication that the circulation of blood is decreasing to the body's extremities and being reserved for the most vital organs. Keep the person warm with a blanket, but do not use one that is electric.

Sleeping

The person may spend an increasing amount of time sleeping, and appear to be uncommunicative or unresponsive and at times be difficult to arouse. This normal change is due in part to changes in the metabolism of the body. Sit with your loved one, hold his or her hand, but do not shake it or speak loudly. Speak softly and naturally. Plan to spend time with your loved one during those times when he or she seems most alert or awake. Do not talk about the person in the person's presence. Speak to him or her directly as you normally would, even though there may be no response. Never assume the person cannot hear; hearing is the last of the senses to be lost.

Disorientation

The person may seem to be confused about the time, place, and identity of people surrounding him or her including close and familiar people. This is also due in part to the metabolism changes. Identify yourself by name before you speak rather than to ask the person to guess who you are. Speak softly, clearly, and truthfully when you need to communicate something important for the patient's comfort, such as, It is time to take your medication, and explain the reason for the communication, such as, so you won't begin to hurt. Do not use this method to try to manipulate the patient to meet your needs.

Incontinence

The person may lose control of urine and/or bowel matter as the muscles in that area begin to relax. Discuss with your Hospice nurse what can be done to protect the bed and keep your loved one clean and comfortable.

Congestion

The person may have gurgling sounds coming from his or her chest as though marbles were rolling around inside these sounds may become very loud. This normal change is due to the decrease of fluid intake and an inability to cough up normal secretions. Suctioning usually only increases the secretions and causes sharp discomfort. Gently turn the person s head to the side and allow gravity to drain the secretions. You may also gently wipe the mouth with a moist cloth. The sound of the congestion does not indicate the onset of severe or new pain.

Restlessness

The person may make restless and repetitive motions such as pulling at bed linen or clothing. This often happens and is due in part to the decrease in oxygen circulation to the brain and to metabolism changes. Do not interfere with or try to restrain such motions. To have a calming effect, speak in a quiet, natural way, lightly massage the forehead, read to the person, or play some soothing music.

Urine Decrease

The person's urine output normally decreases and may become tea colored referred to as concentrated urine. This is due to the decreased fluid intake as well as decrease in circulation through the kidneys. Consult with your Hospice nurse to determine whether there may be a need to insert or irrigate a catheter.

Fluid and Food Decrease

The person may have a decrease in appetite and thirst, wanting little or no food or fluid. The body will naturally begin to conserve energy which is expended on these tasks. Do not try to force food or drink into the person, or try to use guilt to manipulate them into eating or drinking something. To do this only makes the person much more uncomfortable. Small chips of ice, frozen Gatorade or juice may be refreshing in the mouth. If the person is able to swallow, fluids may be given in small amounts by syringe (ask the Hospice nurse for guidance). Glycerin swabs may help keep the mouth and lips moist and comfortable. A cool, moist washcloth on the forehead may also increase physical comfort.

Breathing Pattern Change

The person s regular breathing pattern may change with the onset of a different breathing pace. A particular pattern consists of breathing irregularly, i.e., shallow breaths with periods of no breathing of five to thirty seconds and up to a full minute. This is called Cheyne-Stokes breathing. The person may also experience periods of rapid shallow pant-like breathing. These patterns are very common and indicate decrease in circulation in the internal organs. Elevating the head, and/or turning the person onto his or her side may bring comfort. Hold your loved one's hand. Speak gently.

Withdrawal Normal Emotional, Spiritual, and Mental Signs and Symptoms with Appropriate Responses:

Withdrawal The person may seem unresponsive, withdrawn, or in a comatose-like state. This indicates preparation for release, a detaching from surroundings and relationships, and a beginning of letting go. Since hearing remains all the way to the end, speak to your loved one in your normal tone of voice, identifying yourself by name when you speak, hold his or her hand, and say whatever you need to say that will help the person let go.

Vision-like Experiences

The person may speak or claim to have spoken to persons who have already died, or to see or have seen places not presently accessible or visible to you. This does not indicate an hallucination or a drug reaction. The person is beginning to detach from this life and is being prepared for the transition so it will not be frightening. Do not contradict, explain away, belittle or argue about what the person claims to have seen or heard. Just because you cannot see or hear it does not mean it is not real to your loved one. Affirm his or her experience. They are normal and common. If they frighten your loved one, explain that they are normal occurrences.

Restlessness

The person may perform repetitive and restless tasks. This may in part indicate that something still unresolved or unfinished is disturbing him or her, and prevents him or her from letting go. Your Hospice team members will assist you in identifying what may be happening, and help you find ways to help the person find release from the tension or fear. Other things which may be helpful in calming the person are to recall a favorite place the person enjoyed, a favorite experience, read something comforting, play music, and give assurance that it is OK to let go.

Fluid and Food Decrease

When the person may want little or no fluid or food; this may indicate readiness for the final shut down. Do not try to force food or fluid. You may help your loved one by giving permission to let go whenever he or she is ready. At the same time affirm the person s ongoing value to you and the good you will carry forward into your life that you received from him or her.

Decreased Socialization

The person may only want to be with a very few or even just one person. This is a sign of preparation for release and affirms from whom the support is most needed in order to make the appropriate transition. If you are not part of this inner circle at the end, it does not mean you are not loved or are unimportant. It means you have already fulfilled your task with your loved one, and it is the time for you to say Good-bye. If you are part of the final inner circle of support, the person needs your affirmation, support, and permission.

Unusual Communication

The person may make a seemingly out of character or non sequitur statement, gesture, or request. This indicates that he or she is ready to say Good-bye and is testing you to see if you are ready to let him or her go. Accept the moment as a beautiful gift when it is offered. Kiss, hug, hold, cry, and say whatever you most need to say.

Giving Permission

Giving permission to your loved one to let go, without making him or her guilty for leaving or trying to keep him or her with you to meet your own needs, can be difficult. A dying person will normally try to hold on, even though it brings prolonged discomfort, in order to be sure those who are going to be left behind will be all right. Therefore, your ability to release the dying person from this concern and give him or her assurance that it is all right to let go whenever he or she is ready is one of the greatest gifts you have to give your loved one at this time.

Saying Good-bye

When the person is ready to die and you are able to let go, then is the time to say good-bye. Saying good-bye is your final gift of love to your loved one, for it achieves closure and makes the final release possible.

It may be helpful to lay (sic) in bed and hold the person, or to take his or her hand and then say everything you need to say. It may be as simple as saying, I love you. It may include recounting favorite memories, places, and activities you shared. It may include saying, I 'm sorry for whatever I contributed to any tension or difficulties in our relationship. It may also include saying, Thank you for . . . Tears are a normal and natural part of saying good-bye. Tears do not need to be hidden from your loved one or apologized for. Tears express your love and help you to let go.

How Will You Know When Death Has Occurred?

Although you may be prepared for the death process, you may not be prepared for the actual death moment. It may be helpful for you and your family to think about and discuss what you would do if you were the one present at the death moment. The death of a Hospice patient is not an emergency. Nothing must be done immediately.

The signs of death include such things as no breathing, no heartbeat, release of bowel and bladder, no response, eyelids slightly open, pupils enlarged, eyes fixed on a certain spot, no blinking, jaw relaxed and mouth slightly open. A Hospice nurse will come to assist you if needed or desired. If not, phone support is available.

The body does not have to be moved until you are ready. If the family wants to assist in preparing the body by bathing or dressing, that may be done. Call the funeral home when you are ready to have the body moved, and identify the person as a Hospice patient. The police do not need to be called. The Hospice nurse will notify the physician.

Thank you

We of Hospice thank you for the privilege of assisting you with the care of your loved one. We salute you for all you have done to surround your loved one with understanding care, to provide your loved one with comfort and calm, and to enable your loved one to leave this world with a special sense of peace and love.

You have given your loved one of the most wonderful, beautiful, and sensitive gifts we humans have to offer, and in giving that gift have given yourself a wonderful gift as well.

Related Articles:

Saying Good-bye

Keeping Watch

Stages of Grieving: Death / Dying

From Wikipedia, the free encyclopedia

The Kübler-Ross model, commonly known as the **five stages of grief,** was first introduced by Elisabeth Kübler-Ross in her 1969 book, *On Death and Dying.* [1]It describes, in five discrete stages, a process by which people deal with grief and tragedy, especially when diagnosed with a terminal illness or catastrophic loss. In addition to this, her book brought mainstream awareness to the sensitivity required for better treatment of individuals who are dealing with a fatal disease.[2]

- 1 Stages
- 2 Cultural relevance
- 3 Criticism
- 4 References
- 5 Further reading
- 6 External links

Stages: The progression of states is:[2]   *Wikipedia Free encyclopedia*

1. **Denial** —"I feel fine."; "This can't be happening, not to me. "Denial is usually only a temporary defense for the individual. This feeling is generally replaced with heightened awareness of situations and individuals that will be left behind after death.

2. **Anger** —"Why me? It's not fair!"; "How can this happen to me?"; *"Who is to blame?"* Once in the second stage, the individual recognizes that denial cannot continue. Because of anger, the person is very difficult to care for due to misplaced feelings of rage and envy. Any individual that symbolizes life or energy is subject to projected resentment and jealousy.

3. **Bargaining**—"Just let me live to see my children graduate."; "I'll do anything for a few more years."; "I will give my life savings if . . ."

109

4. The third stage involves the hope that the individual can somehow postpone or delay death. Usually, the negotiation for an extended life is made with a higher power in exchange for a reformed lifestyle. Psychologically, the individual is saying, "I understand I will die, but if I could just have more time . . ."

5. **Depression** —"I'm so sad, why bother with anything?"; "I'm going to die . . . What's the point?"; "I miss my loved one, why go on?" During the fourth stage, the dying person begins to understand the certainty of death. Because of this, the individual may become silent, refuse visitors and spend much of the time crying and grieving. This process allows the dying person to disconnect oneself from things of love and affection. It is not recommended to attempt to cheer up an individual who is in this stage. It is an important time for grieving that must be processed.

6. **Acceptance** —"It's going to be okay."; "I can't fight it, I may as well prepare for it." This final stage comes with peace and understanding of the death that is approaching. Generally, the person in the fifth stage will want to be left alone. Additionally, feelings and physical pain may be non-existent. This stage has also been described as the end of the dying struggle.

Kübler-Ross originally applied these stages to people suffering from terminal illness, later to any form of catastrophic personal loss (job, income, freedom). This may also include significant life events such as the death of a loved one, divorce, drug addiction, an infertility diagnosis, as well many tragedies and disasters.

Kübler-Ross claimed these steps do not necessarily come in the order noted above, nor are all steps experienced by all patients, though she stated a person will always experience at least two. Often, people will experience several stages in a "roller coaster" effect—switching between two or more stages, returning to one or more several times before working through it.[2]

Significantly, people experiencing the stages should not force the process. The grief process is highly personal and should not be rushed, nor lengthened, on the basis of an individual's imposed time frame or opinion. One should merely be aware that the stages will be worked through and the ultimate stage of "Acceptance" will be reached.

However, there are individuals who struggle with death until the end. Some psychologists believe that the harder a person fights death, the more likely they are to stay in the denial stage. If this is the case, it is possible the ill person will have more difficulty dying in a dignified way. Other psychologists state that not confronting death until the end is adaptive for some people.[2] Those who experience problems working through the stages should consider professional grief counseling or support groups.

Cultural relevance

A dying individual's approach to death has been linked to the amount of meaning and purpose a person has found throughout their lifetime. A study of 160 people with less than three months to live showed that those who felt they understood their purpose in life, or found special meaning, faced less fear and despair in the final weeks of their lives than those who had not. In this and similar studies, spirituality helped dying individuals deal with the depression stage more aggressively than those who were not spiritual. [2]

Author's Comment: A convenient way to remember Dr. Kubler Ross' Stages of Death and Dying would be to use the acronym DABDA, i.e.

D = *Denial; A= Anger; B* = *Bargaining; D* = *Depression; A* = *Acceptance*

This article uses bare URLs in its references. Please use proper citations containing each referenced work's title, author, date, and source, so that the article remains verifiable in the future.

Help may be available. Several templates are available for formatting. (March 2010)

1. ^ "Milestones". TIME. Aug. 30, 2004. http://www.time. com/time/magazine/article/0,9171,689491,00.html.
2. ^ *a b c d e* Santrock, J.W. (2007). *A Topical Approach to Life-Span Development*. New York: McGraw-Hill. ISBN 0073382647.
3. ^ http://www.tc.columbia.edu/faculty/index. htm?facid=gab38 George A. Bonanno's Columbia University Faculty Page
4. ^ Bonanno, George (2009). *The Other Side of Sadness: What the New Science of Bereavement Tells Us About Life After a Loss*. Basic Books. ISBN 9780465013609. http://www.perseusbooksgroup.com/basic/book detail. jsp?isbn=0465013600.
5. ^ Maciejewski, P.K., *JAMA* (February 21, 2007). Retrieved April 14, 2009, http://jama.ama-assn.org/cgi/ content/abstract/297/7/716?etoc
6. ^ Friedman and James. "The Myth of the Stages of Dying, Death and Grief", *Skeptic Magazine* (2008). Retrieved 2008, from http://www.grief.net/Articles/Myth%20 of%20Stages.pdf

Further reading

- Kübler-Ross, E. (1973) *On Death and Dying*, Routledge, ISBN 0415040159
- Kübler-Ross, E. (2005) *On Grief and Grieving: Finding the Meaning of Grief Through the Five Stages of Loss*, Simon & Schuster Ltd, ISBN 0743263448
- Scire, P. (2007). "Applying Grief Stages to Organizational Change"
- *An Attributional Analysis of Kübler-Ross' Model of Dying*, Mark R Brent. Harvard University, 1981.

- *An Evaluation of the Relevance of the Kübler-Ross Model to the Post-injury Responses of Competitive Athletes,* Johannes Hendrikus Van der Poel, University of the Free State. Published by s.n., 2000.

External links

- Elisabeth Kübler-Ross Homepage
- Elisabeth Kübler-Ross—five stages of grief
- *On Death and Dying*—Interview With Elizabeth Kübler-Ross M.D.
- *Beware the Five Stages of Grief*—TLC Group Editorial

Retrieved from "http://en.wikipedia.org/wiki/K%C3%BCbler-Ross model"
Categories: 1969 books | Grief | Psychiatry works | Psychological theories | Psychology books | Self-help books

Interaction

- About Wikipedia
- Contact Wikipedia
- This page was last modified on 29 April 2010 at 13:44.
- Text is available under the Creative Commons Attribution-ShareAlike License; additional terms may apply. See Terms of Use for details.
- Wikipedia® is a registered trademark of the Wikimedia Foundation, Inc., a non-profit organization.

CHAPTER 12

WHO PAYS FOR HOSPICE BENEFITS?

The Federal Government has determined that Hospice Care is an established part of the overall healthcare system. Therefore the costs for providing Hospice Care Services are covered and paid for by Medicare Benefits.

If a patient is a Medicare beneficiary the Hospice Benefits are covered under Part A. other Hospice services are covered under Parts A and B including payment to the Primary or Attending Physician.

At this writing—as of 2006, *the latest figures available*—46 states and the District of Columbia offered Hospice Care coverage as a Medicaid Benefit. Medicaid is a state and federal partnership designed to offer health care for people with low-incomes who otherwise might not be able to receive health care benefits.

Medicaid is a state controlled program made available to certain low-income individuals and families who must meet certain eligibility group criteria recognized by both federal and state law. Medicaid is administered by individual states and each state sets its own guide lines with regard to eligibility and services.

Individuals who are medically needy with low-incomes may become eligible for Medicaid benefits due to the low-income and excessive medical expenses.

If you or a loved one have low-income, with a terminal illness diagnosis, and a life expectancy of less than 6 months and have been recommend by your Primary or Attending Physician to become a hospice patient, you may be eligible for Medicaid benefits. Even if you are unsure you qualify you should have a qualified hospice Medical Social Worker evaluate your situation.

Some private insurance health care plans have a hospice benefit provision for its members. A check with the private insurance company representative would enable the inquirer to obtain this information.

NOTE: This Hospice Guide Book contains rules and regulations which were legally in force at the time of this writing. State and federal regulations, rules and laws may change with implementation of the Health Care Reform Bill passed in March 2010.

CHAPTER 13

WHO IS ELIGIBLE FOR HOSPICE CARE?

- Q. When can a patient go on to a Hospice program?

- A. If a medical doctor diagnoses a patient's disease as terminal, with less than six months to live, they become eligible for Hospice care. This applies to anyone who has been diagnosed with a terminal illness with a six month Or less life expectancy.

  Any patient in the final stages of life is eligible; there is no age restriction.

- Q. What happens if a patient's condition improves?

- A. If a patient's health improves and Hospice is no longer needed, the patient can refuse further Hospice care.

- Q. If a patient's health declines can they get back on Hospice?

- *A.* Yes. A patient is eligible to reapply for Hospice if necessary.

- Q. Can a patient go into the hospital when on Hospice?

- A. Yes. If the hospitalization is not related to the Hospice diagnosis, and the hospitalization is to improve the patient's quality of life, i.e. comfort care.

- **Q.** Is Hospice only for patients with cancer disease terminal illness?

- **A. No. Patients diagnosed with other terminal illness diseases can also be**

- **Q.** Does a patient have to give up Hospice if they go into a nursing home?

- **A. No. Not if the Hospice agency has a contract agreement with the nursing home allowing the Interdisciplinary Group (IDG) team to provide the primary care.**

- **Q.** When a patient chooses Hospice care do they have to stay in hospice until they die?

- **A. No. A patient can change their mind and seek aggressive, curative treatment at any time; a patient can choose to go on, and off hospice care as needed.**

- **Q.** Does Medicare pay regardless of where the patient resides?

- **A. No. Medicare requires Hospice care to be provided at the home residence.**

- **Medicare does pay for short term facility admissions for in-patient and respite care**

- **Q.** Does a patient choosing Hospice give up the right to curative care treatment?

- **A. Yes. The patient has elected to choose comfort, rather than aggressive care.**

CHAPTER 14

IS HOSPICE CARE FOR YOU OR A LOVED ONE?

Hospice is not a "One size fits all," program. Neither will it serve to satisfy the demands and requirements of every individual who is diagnosed with a terminal illness.

The decision in giving consent to be admitted into a Hospice program needs to be carefully weighed by asking multiple, first person, singular questions.

For example:

What did my doctor say? Was I diagnosed with a life-limiting, terminal illness?

Is my condition really irreversible? Or should I pursue aggressive treatment?

If I choose not to pursue aggressive treatment, what is the length of my life expectancy?

Will I die in pain? Or, will my symptoms be well managed?

What are my options? Can I choose to stay in my home? Who will take care of me?

What will my quality of life be like if I choose hospice?

Will I be abandoned and left alone to die?

Will I be able to call "911?

Will I be able to go to the hospital if needed?

What about concerns I might have, other than pain, or symptom control? Such as, depression; fears, spiritual needs, etc.

All these areas of concern are important to a prospective hospice patient and need to be addressed and discussed with a knowledgeable Hospice representative.

While many of these concerns and questions are dealt with in other chapters of this publication, A Hospice Guide Book, and they will be highlighted and discussed briefly again here, in the order presented.

Q. What did my doctor say? Was I diagnosed with a life-limiting, terminal illness?

    A.   **If your doctor has diagnosed you with a terminal illness, with a life expectancy of 6 months or less, your disease has reached the final stages.**

Q. Is my condition really irreversible? Or should I pursue aggressive treatment?

    A.   **When a patient is diagnosed with a terminal illness the disease has progressed to the irreversible stage and does not usually respond to aggressive treatment.**

Q. If I choose not to pursue aggressive treatment, what is the length of my life expectancy?

A. No one can accurately determine the exact length of life expectancy. The 6 months or less life expectancy, required by Hospice regulations, is based on on statistical averages.

Q. Will I die in pain? Or, will my symptoms be well managed?

A. No. One of the key elements in receiving Hospice care is the excellent pain and symptom management control.

Q. What are my options? Can I choose to stay in my home? Who will take care of me?

A. When a patient exercise the option to enter a Hospice program they usually stay in their own home, surrounded by loved ones and a familiar environment. Many Hospice patients are cared for by family members who serve as Primary Caregivers (PCG's)

Q. What will my quality of life be like if I choose Hospice?

A. The goal of Hospice is to provide the best quality of life possible 7/24/365.

Q. Will I be abandoned and left alone to die?

A. As long as a patient qualifies, and chooses to stay in a hospice program, they are cared for by a team of professionals, Nurses, Social Workers, Chaplains, and Volunteers who are dedicated to providing on-going, medical, psychosocial, spiritual counseling, nurturing support.

Q. Will I be able to call "911? Will I be able to go to the hospital if needed?

A. **Hospice patient or family member is never prohibited from calling "911." Yes. You can go to a hospital; however, hospice care is designed to avoid frequent hospitalizations by treating the patients pain and symptoms at home.**

Other issues and questions can, and will, be discussed, and answered, at patient request, by a qualified Hospice Benefits Admission Coordinator.

CHAPTER 15

MAKING THE RIGHT DECISION

Patients and families often need professional counsel and guidance when making a decision whether or not Hospice Care is appropriate, and the right choice for them.

The question: Is Hospice the right choice? Making a decision to enroll in, and be admitted to a hospice program, can be a highly emotional, difficult, and sometimes frightening experience. The patient has to make a decision, to move from a curative modality of treatment of the disease, to a palliative, or comfort care stage. In other words, forming a new mindset of adjusting to and accepting the terminal illness, and the 6 month life expectancy, instead of fighting it with aggressive treatment in the hope of obtaining a cure.

Hospice care is appropriate, when the patient's physician informs the patient that the terminal disease has advanced beyond a point of no return, to where a curative modality of treatment is no longer indicated, and further curative measures would fail to produce positive results.

Whereas. The curative modality focused on aggressive treatment, in an attempt to cure the disease. On the other hand, comfort care, or the palliative care model, focuses solely on providing patient symptom management, pain control, and providing support for the family.

After being diagnosed with a terminal illness, and referred by a medical doctor to Hospice Care, the patient is faced with a major decision; anticipation in making a decision presents many questions.

For example:

Q. Should I, or shouldn't I, make a decision? This is a very important decision. It is a life-changing decision. When is the appropriate time? If there is only six months life expectancy, do I need to make a decision right away?

A. From a medical perspective, a patient is immediately faced with making decision, after their doctor tells them they have a terminal illness with less than a six month life expectancy. It is also at this time the medical doctor will counsel with the patient that it is no longer reasonable to continue with life-sustaining treatment.

To delay, or put off the decision, is to deny the patient the benefit of receiving the care from a team of trained supportive professionals, and of spending the last part of their lives comfortably, and free from pain.

Too often, a decision to enter into a Hospice program is delayed until the patient is within days of dying; when patients wait too long to take advantage of the Hospice Benefit Program, valuable time is lost, and the patient becomes unable to cognitively communicate with loved ones, or to appreciate the care and comfort care measures for symptom management, and pain control.

Once a decision has been made to pursue Hospice Care the Interdisciplinary Group (IDG) team will be put in place, and Hospice services will commence, for medical, psychosocial, spiritual, counselors, and volunteers will commence. A Plan of Care (POC) will be developed, uniquely tailored to each patient's needs and wishes.

Q. What happens if a decision is made to pursue Aggressive Treatment?

A. A patient can choose to revoke, and leave the Hospice program, at any time. If a patient revokes, and then decides to re-enter the hospice program, they can again be re-admitted.

NOTE: Hospice admission professionals are readily available, through the patients'/families Hospice agency of choice, to answer any/all questions about Hospice Care and services. In the Hospice local office, or in the patient's home—specific issues relating to the patient, family and caregivers—will be discussed with family, and care givers present. By having spouses, a family member, and caregivers present, ensures inclusion and involvement in the patient's Hospice Care.

GLOSSARY

This Glossary of definitions and terms is not inclusive; it is primarily Hospice specific, although, there are terms which are also generic to healthcare and medical care, the terms are not intended to offer medical advice and / or diagnosis, or be definitive of all symptoms, diseases and / or illnesses.

Rather, it is intended to give an overall general brief definition of the subject matter. Patients and family members seeking medical advice and information, with regard to disease symptoms and or illness, should contact their own medical doctor professionals.

A

Activities of Daily Living (ADL's): Refers to normal self-activities done in daily living.

Acute Care: Care usually received in a hospital for acute illness, injury or surgery recovery.

Admission: The acceptance and entry of a patient into any kind of medical treatment.

Admission Registered Nurse (RN): Nurses who provide patient admission for medical treatment.

Admitting Physician: The physician responsible for admitting a patient for medical treatment.

Advance Directive: Two kinds of documents; Medical (Durable) Power of Attorney, and Living Wills. Provides direction to surrogate (an appointed person), about future medical treatments wanted on behalf of the patient in case of patient incapacity.

Against Medical Advice (AMA): Refers to a patient that checks themselves out of a treatment center against the advice of their doctor.

Aging: The process of becoming older experienced by all.

Ambulatory: Able to walk around with or without assistance.

Ancillary Services: Services provided for X-Rays and / or laboratory tests.

Assessment: Evaluation a patient's health status through physical or mental examination, combined with review of patient medical history.

Authorization: The patient's health plan usually requires authorization be given prior to a doctor performing surgery or extensive medical procedures.

Attending Physician aka **Primary Care Physician**: The doctor responsible for the total medical care of a patient.

B

Benefit Penalty: When the rules of the health plan are not specifically followed a penalty usually occurs.

Bereavement: To be in a lonely or sad state of mind due to acute loss or death of a loved one; characterized by emotional, behavioral, and physical changes.

Bereavement Counselor: Usually, but not always, a clergy person offering counseling to the surviving bereaved during a time of loss or death of a loved one.

C

Caregivers: An individual, either paid professional or volunteer, who provides care and assistance usually in the home to aging, terminally ill, or disabled persons.

Care Plan: Established by each professional team member, a Plan of Care (POC) details the level of care, the medical and physical treatment to be performed on the patient, the frequency of the treatment, and by whom the treatment will be given.

Case Manager: In hospice care the term usually refers to the Registered Nurse (RN) assigned to the patient who monitors the patient's medical needs, controls their pain, and manages all of the patient's symptoms.

Center of Disease Control (CDC): A federal agency controlled by the United States Department of Health and Human Services. Located in Atlanta, Georgia its function is to provide public health and safety measures by networking with state and private health organizations.

Certification: A term used to describe the process for certifying an individual applying for benefits under a particular medical program; certification indicates that all criteria has been met and that the applying individual is eligible for certification.

Certified Nursing Assistant (CAN): An trained professional individual who assists patient's with health care needs to include, but not limited to, basic nursing procedures working under the supervision of a Registered Nurse (RN).

Chaplain: A clergyperson who provides pastoral and spiritual care and counsel to patients and families struggling with religious issues. Chaplains are always available to assist families and care givers, after the death of a loved one, with bereavement counseling, funeral and memorial services.

Charity Care: Medicare law provides that no person may be refused hospice care due to inability to pay. Financial analysts are available through hospice agencies for consultation and counsel with patients and families about receiving financial assistance.

Clinical Social Worker aka Medical Social Worker: A professional licensed social worker who assess and evaluates a patient's ability to live independently, or with a primary caregiver, in a home environment; develops a Plan of Care (POC) for needed and necessary home services, frequency of visits, and needed durable medical equipment.

Cognitive: Possession of a sharp mind that is able to reason and think clearly, and respond appropriately to interaction, with the ability to make proper decisions; the ability to choose between right and wrong.

Certified Home Health Aide *aka* **Bath Aide***:*

The Certified Home Health Aides aka Bath Aide, and Home Health Aide, is a very important member of the Hospice and / or home health care team, who helps the patient to retain confidence and independent. Their daily/weekly routine duties include, but are not limited to the following:

Assist the patient with bathing; in-bed, shower or tub, and their toileting

To help with care of teeth, mouth, and oral hygiene

To aid with transfer of patient from bed to chair, chair to wheelchair, and in walking

Assist with grooming: hair, care of nails (not toenails), *and male patients* electric shaving

To aid in dressing the patient

If present at mealtime to help with serving nutrition and aiding patient feed self

To assist by providing patient overall hygiene

Assist patient with Durable Medical Equipment, safety and mobility, e.g. wheel chairs, Hoyer Lifts, Walkers, etc.

Remind patients to take medications on time (to be dispensed / given by family members

Confidentiality: To maintain a patient's privacy and confidentiality, with regard to patient information i.e. medical history and medical records, and to share that information only with individuals, companies and organizations *that have a right to know that information.*

Competence: Usually refers to the patient's mental status and alertness, i.e. the patient knows who they are, where they are, and why they are there in that location. This is referred to as a patient being A/O X's 3. Other tools used to determine competence is asking questions like: Who is the President of the U.S.? What year is this? What Month, day, etc.?

Continuous Quality Improvement (CQI): The Quality Improvement Manager directs and manages continuing hospice / health care Quality Assurance Performance Improvement (QAPI) activity movement to assure compliance with all federal Medicare laws, state regulations, and local laws including responsibility to monitor and facilitates performance achievement through a compilation of local, state, and national data analysis, to include satisfaction surveys, clinical record reviews, and comparative scores.

D

Deductible: The fixed amount a patient must pay prior to an insurance plan paying benefits; aka as co-pay.

Depression: A state of mind illness condition which involves the body, mind, mood, and thought process affecting eating, feelings, thinking and actions. Untreated symptoms can be long-lasting and can result in suicidal ideations. With appropriate treatment of symptoms, depression can be controlled with psychotropic medication, and most people can be helped to cope appropriately.

Designation of Health Care Surrogate aka **Durable Power of Attorney**: A legal document appointing another person, usually a family member, to make medical decision for the patient, if the patient is incapacitated, and unable to make decisions for themselves.

Diagnosis (DX): This is the term applied by a medical doctor to a patient's disease condition consistent with assessed evidence of standard and accepted medical diagnostic criteria signs and symptoms.

Discharge: The release of a patient under medical care from a healthcare facility, hospital or course of medical treatment.

DNR: Order Verification Form: A medical doctor's written orders to healthcare providers—at the request of patient or family members—that a patient is not to receive cardiopulmonary resuscitation (CPR) in the event of cardiac arrest (heart stoppage). In order to be legally valid the DNR must be signed by a physician.

DNR: Order Verification Protocol: This document directs Emergency Medical Service (EMS) personnel, paramedics and first responders that a patient in cardiac or respiratory distress will not receive resuscitative measures, rather, that the patient is only to receive palliative comfort care.

Durable Medical Equipment (DME): Medical equipment used in the care and treatment of home patients to include, but not limited to, crutches, hospital beds, oxygen concentrators / tanks supplies, walkers, wheelchairs, etc.

Durable Power of Attorney (Health): A legal document designating another person to make health decisions for the patient if the patient is incapacitated and unable to make decisions for themselves. (See also Advance Directive)

Durable Power of Attorney (General): A general Power of Attorney is used to allow an appointed agent all business, financial, legal, or other affairs during a period of time when the individual / patient is incapacitated and unable to do so.

E

Emergency Medical services (EMS): Both government and private Agencies which provide medical services usually outside of healthcare by facilities.

Emergency Medical Technician (EMT): Medical personnel trained in the procedures required in the performance of emergency care.

Emergency Room (ER): A room set aside in acute care facilities or hospitals to receive patients transported by ambulance or Paramedics who are severely injured, traumatized, seriously ill or have experienced a heart attack or repository distress.

End-of Life Comfort Care / Palliative Care Hospice: Medical care designed to control pain and manage symptoms, and to improve the quality of life for a patient who has a life-limiting illness or terminal disease.

End-Stage Renal Disease (ESRD): Refers to kidney disease and failure of kidney's to even respond to dialysis; failure diseased of kidneys that have totally stopped functioning.

Ethics: Discussion and Consideration of: Principles and values that guide ethical decision making and conduct based on medical facts.

Explanation of Benefits (EOB): Providing an explanation of benefits (especially in hospice) to patients / families considering hospice care as a medical alternative.

F No entry

G

Grief: The act of reacting to a loss (divorce), occupational (loss of employment), or physical death of a loved one. Anxiety and stress caused by grief can affect eating, sleeping, bodily functioning, and illness.

Grief Support Center: Bereavement Programs set up by hospitals, hospice agencies, and civic organizations offering grief and bereavement net-working meetings in support of patient survivors.

Guardianship: An individual who has been legally appointed and authorized to act for another person, who has been judged to be mentally incompetent, and to make both medical and fiduciary decisions on behalf of that person, who is unable to act on their own behalf.

H

Hospice: A program designed to provide palliative care, aka, comfort care, usually in a home setting, for patients who have been diagnosed with a terminal illness and are near the end of their life.

Hospice Agency: A free-standing medical office facility acting as an agency to admit and provide palliative aka comfort care for terminally ill patients; funded by either Medicare or Medicaid benefit programs

Hospice Provider: The term describes ancillary services, usually private (can be public) companies or agencies contracted by the hospice agency, providing hospice organizations portable radiation units, X-ray service, and laboratory testing.

Hospice Team: A team of professionals to include, Medical Director (MD); Admissions Coordinator; Patient Care Manager; Admitting Nurse—Registered Nurse (RN); Medical Social Worker (MSW); Chaplain; Certified Home Health Aide (CHHA); Bereavement Coordinator (BC);, and Volunteer Coordinator.

Health Care Directive: A patient's legal document completed while the patient was alert, aware, and cognitive, stating whether the patient would want to remain on life sustaining support in the event they become comatose, unable to speak for themselves.

Health Insurance Portability and Accountability Act (HIPPA): The acronym stands for Health Insurance Portability and Accountability Act (HIPPA 1996, i.e., HIPPA Policy 6.1. Strict rules and regulations are in place regarding patient privacy and confidentiality. Violations are legally and stringently enforced with stringent penalties, imposed by both civil **and criminal courts.**

From Wikipedia, the free encyclopedia

The **Health Insurance Portability and Accountability Act (HIPAA) of 1996 (P.L.104-191)** [**HIPAA**] was enacted by the U.S. Congress in 1996. It was originally sponsored by Sen. Edward Kennedy (D-Mass.) and Sen. Nancy Kassebaum (R-Kan.). According to the Centers for Medicare and Medicaid Services (CMS) website, Title I of HIPAA protects health insurance coverage for workers and their families when they change or lose their jobs. Title II of HIPAA, known as the Administrative Simplification (AS) provisions, requires the establishment of national standards for electronic health care transactions and national identifiers for providers, health insurance plans, and employers.

The Administration Simplification provisions also address the security and privacy of health data. The standards are meant to improve the efficiency and effectiveness of the nation's health care system by encouraging the widespread use of electronic data interchange in the U.S. health care system

Health Maintenance Organization (HMO): A healthcare organization provider system employing medical professionals to provide specific medical services to members of the (HMO) who are pre-paid subscribers.

Health Care Management Systems (HPMS): A data base of current eligible and enrolled patients who are recipients of Medicare Parts A and Part B.

I

Independent Living: The term describes an individual who resides in a senior housing setting providing supportive services such as, housekeeping, laundry, meals, social activities and transportation to and from doctor appointments.

Informed Consent: The assurance of professional disclosure, and patient understanding, of medical information, and their willingness and competent ability to be able to cognitively consent to medical procedures.

EXCEPTION: Emergency Conditions: Under the law, doctors and medical personnel are legally and morally obligated—*except in emergency situations*—to obtain a patient's informed consent prior to performing any invasive medical procedures.

Interdisciplinary Group (IDG) Team: A team of skilled professionals, health care providers (especially in hospice care), composed of a Medical Director, Patient Care Manger, Registered Nurse (RN) Case Manager, Medical Social Worker (MSW), Chaplain, Bereavement Coordinator, Volunteer Coordinator and volunteer, who provide both medical and supportive services to a patient through the end-of-life process.

Intensive Care: Intense, continuous care provided to critically ill patients by trained medical professional doctors and nurses in an acute hospital ward, called the Intensive Care Unit (ICU).

Initial Nursing Assessment (INA): Usually the first nursing visit to a patient after they have been admitted to medical treatment / care (especially in hospice). It is during this assessment that the patient's medical needs are evaluated and a Plan of Care (POC) protocol is established for treatment modality, medications, and frequency of visits.

L

Length of Stay (LOS): Refers to the time frame for length of stay, from admission to discharge; the number of day, weeks, etc. that a patient is confined for treatment in a hospital or medical facility.

Level of Care: Refers to the intensity for medical care treatment for a patient admitted to a hospital or medical facility.

Life-Limiting Illness: An illness that does not respond to cure oriented medical treatment, aka aggressive treatment; (in hospice) an disease which has been diagnosed as a terminal illness.

Long-term Care: Services usually provided (in hospice) at home; or in an assisted living environment; in a skilled nursing facility (SNF) or nursing home, aka long term care center (LTCC), provided for both hospice and chronically ill patients who can no longer care for themselves.

M

Medical Director: In hospice, a Medical Doctor is usually trained in the specialty of cancer (oncology), and end-of-life disease treatments, i.e. comfort care, palliative care as well as general medical practice; responsible for overall patient medical treatment to ensure the highest quality standard of professional medical care.

Medicare: An established federal government health care program, passed by Congress for persons 65 years and older, and the disabled, who are Social Security Medicare recipients, to provide medical insurance payment to eligible participants for medical treatment received.

Medicare Part A: Medicare Insurance that pays for hospice benefits and in-patient stays for hospital and Skilled Nursing Facility (SNF's), and partial healthcare coverage.

Medicare Part B: Medicare Insurance that pays for doctor visits, Durable Medical Equipment (DME), and laboratory tests to include some medical treatment services.

Medicare Advantage: An alternative to Part A, and Part B healthcare coverage provided Patients by private companies.

Medicaid: This is a state program designed to offer public assistance to persons whose income and resources are not sufficient to pay for health care, regardless of age. The federal government provides matching funds to help finance the state Medicaid program.

Medical Records Number (MD#): This refers to the identification number assigned to a patient's Medical Record aka Patient's Medical Record Chart.

N

Nursing Home: Nursing Home aka Skilled Nursing Facility (SNF), typically involves providing and managing complex and / or potentially serious medical issues to include, but not limited to, coma care, tube feeding, infections, wound care, and IV Therapy. Both short term and long term care is provided for those with serious medical problems and disabilities and others who are bedbound, wheelchair bound, totally non-ambulatory and are need dependent for all Activities of Daily Living (ADL's), with maximum assist. Typically, Nursing Home Care is provided for those patients who have a serious disability to the extent that the services they need cannot be found through residential care, i.e., Nursing Home Care typically involves providing and managing complex and / or potentially serious medical issues to include, but not limited to, coma care, tube feeding, infections, wound care, and IV Therapy.

Both short term and long term care is provided for those with serious medical problems and disabilities and others who are bedbound, wheelchair bound, totally non-ambulatory and are need dependent for all Activities of Daily Living (ADL's), with maximum assist.

Typically, Nursing Home Care is provided for those patients who have a serious disability to the extent that the services they need cannot be found through residential care, i.e., Board and Cares facilities, or home care.

O

On Call (OC): Health care professionals are routinely placed on call (OC) during their regular off-duty hours in order to respond to patient emergency needs.

Ombudsman: A government official who investigates complaints against healthcare facilities in order to improve the resident's quality of life.

Out Patient (OP): Refers to patients who are transported to and from a medical center facility and receive treatment without having to be hospitalized.

P

Palliative Care: Also known as comfort care; medical care / treatment given to patients who have a life-limiting or terminal illness to improve the quality of life.

Pain Management: A term used to describe treatment with medication to control pain and to manage symptoms of pain.

Pastoral Care: The overall spiritual support care, performed by a clergy person through counseling, for patient increased spiritual affirmation, decreased angst, anxiety, isolation, and to provide on-going spiritual visits for patient comfort and encouragement.

Patient Care Manager: The Interdisciplinary Group (IDG) is led by the Patient Care Manager (PCM) who is responsible for coordinating all of the patient's service, and Plan of Care (POC), from the admission start of (SOC) to the patient's death, or other type discharge.

The Patient Care Manager (PCM) attends all Interdisciplinary Group (IDG) meetings and communicates on a regular basis with the patient, and the Registered Nurse (RN) Case Manager, providing a direct link between them, enabling clear communication to freely flow, permitting the exchange of patient information helping them to stay informed about the patient's clinical and medical condition. Both also maintain an "as needed" direct contact with the Medical Director, and pharmacists, to be able to obtain the physician orders and, to obtain the necessary authorization for pain medication, and other medications, plus dieticians, and all other members of the Health Care Team, for ongoing patient care and comfort needs.

Physical Therapy (PT): A trained medical Physical Therapist professional who administers patient range of motion, ambulatory assistance, and treatment to develop and maintain patient maximum movement and motion throughout their life.

Power of Attorney: A Power of Attorney legal documents; Two types: **One**, aka Durable Power of Attorney, provides for Medical Decision making, by another party on behalf of the patient, when the patient is unable to make independent decisions for themselves. **Two**, a General Power of Attorney provides for one person to act in legal matters on another's behalf for financial or real estate transactions.

Primary Care Giver: A relative, friend, or paid professional, who is trained to work closely with medical staff and family members, to provide assistance with reminding the responsible party Durable Power of Attorney for Medical purpose, to give medications, bathing, feeding, and comfort care aka palliative care to chronically ill or end-of-life, terminally ill patients.

Private Duty Nursing Services: Nurses hired through a private agency organization to provide necessary medical services to patients requiring continuous in-homecare that is not immediately obtainable through hospice or a home health agency.

Private Pay: Refers to payments made directly to the medical provider or health care facility by the patient and / or family. This is considered to be an out-of-pocket expense not reimbursed by either a private or public healthcare insurance plan

Q

Quality Assurance (QA): On-going assessment of medical and nursing activities to evaluate and ensure the quality of care being provided.

Quality of Life: An ambiguous term with various meanings, i.e. receiving the right comfort care, control of pain and management of symptoms, all of which contribute to the quality of a patient's life. In fact, and in reality, quality of life is considered to be patient-centered emphasizing self-worth, i.e. the worth of the patient to self.

Quality Management (QM): The on-going evaluation and assessment, to measure and improve, the quality of care being provided by a health care organization.

R

Recertification: A term used to describe the process for re-certifying an individual applying for continuing benefits under a particular medical program; re-certification indicates that all criteria has been met and that the applying individual is eligible for re-certification.

Referral: Refers to any patient or family being referred by another person to an agency or medical facility for hospice or other kinds of medical treatment.

Registered Nurse (RN): The RN Case Manager (in hospice), works closely with the Medical Director and Attending physician to ensure that the patient's medical needs are being appropriately addressed and met, that pain and symptoms are being controlled, and that the patient is kept as free from pain, with needs met, and as comfortable as possible.

Rehabilitation: Rehabilitative therapy and training uniquely designed for specific patients, and provided by a trained healthcare medical professional, to assist a patient recover skills that have been compromised by injury or illness.

Resident Care Coordinator (RCC): Resident Care Coordinators work under the direct supervision of the administrator and responsible to ensure that patients /residents receive the best possible quality of care.

Respiratory Therapy: A therapy to assist and treat patients recover from lung function such as respiratory distress and other acute or chronic breathing disorders

Respite Care: Admittance (maximum 5 days @ a time in hospice) of a hospice patient in a healthcare facility for temporary relief of the Primary Caregivers (PCG) and family members—to give them a break—. from the stress of caregiving. The timeframe can range from 3 to 5 days.

S

Spiritual Care Coordinator (SCC) aka Chaplain: A clergyperson who provides up-lifting comfort, pastoral, spiritual care and counsel to patients and families struggling with religious issues and life-limiting illnesses. Chaplains are always available to assist families and care givers, after the death of a loved one, with bereavement counseling, funeral and memorial services.

Speech Therapy: Usually therapy provided by a trained speech therapist to patients for recovery and rehabilitation of speech that has been compromised by a disease, i.e. Parkinson's disease, a cardiovascular attack (CVA), stroke, or other disease affecting speech.

Start of Care (SOC): Also know as admission; this refers to the date of patient admission to medical care treatment.

Skilled Nursing Facility (SNF) aka Nursing Home: A Skilled Nursing Facility (SNF) aka Nursing Home Care typically involves providing and managing complex and / or potentially serious medical issues to include, but not limited to, coma care, tube feeding, infections, wound care, and IV Therapy. Both short term and long term care is provided for those with serious medical problems and disabilities and others who are bedbound, wheelchair bound, totally non-ambulatory and are need dependent for all Activities of Daily Living (ADL's), with maximum assist. Typically, Nursing Home Care is provided for those patients who have a serious disability to the extent that the services they need cannot be found through residential care, i.e., Nursing Home Care typically involves providing and managing complex and / or potentially serious medical issues to include, but not limited to, coma care, tube feeding, infections, wound care, and IV Therapy. Both short term and long term care is provided for those with serious medical problems and disabilities and others who are bedbound, wheelchair bound, totally non-ambulatory and are need dependent for all Activities of Daily Living (ADL's), with maximum assist. Typically, Nursing Home Care is provided for those patients who have a serious disability to the extent that the services they need cannot be found through residential care, i.e., Board and Cares facilities, or home care.

T

Treatment (TX): This term refers to the treatment modality protocol elected by the Medical Director (MD), attending Physician (MD), and Registered Nurse (RN) Case Manager. The abbreviation acronym TX is used to designate the word treatment.

Third-party Payer: A private or public organization that insures health and medical expenses on behalf of a recipient and pays for medical fees on the patient's behalf.

U

No entry

V

No entry

W

World Health Organization (WHO): An agency under the control of the United Nations designed to enhance cooperation for improvement of health conditions around the world. Its designated stated purpose is to promote "the highest possible level of health," by all people.

X

X-ray: Radiation; purpose is to take images inside of the body through penetration; a photograph made with X-rays.

Y

No Entry

Z

Zone of Comfort: Refers to the state of a patient's on-going mental and physical condition; i.e. freedom from pain, with needs met, and a comfortable status.

Resources

Stages of Grieving: Death / Dying   From Wikipedia, the free
encyclopedia

The Kübler-Ross model, commonly known as the **five stages of grief**, was first introduced by <u>Elisabeth Kübler-Ross</u> in her 1969 book, *On Death and Dying.* [1]It describes, in five discrete stages, a process by which people deal with <u>grief</u> and tragedy, especially when diagnosed with a terminal illness or catastrophic loss. In addition to this, her book brought mainstream awareness to the sensitivity required for better treatment of individuals who are dealing with a fatal disease.[2]

Stages The progression of states is:[2]   **Wikipedia Free encyclopedia**

1. **<u>Denial</u>** —"I feel fine."; "This can't be happening, not to me." Denial is usually only a temporary defense for the individual. This feeling is generally replaced with heightened awareness of situations and individuals that will be left behind after death.
2. **<u>Anger</u>** —"Why me? It's not fair!"; "How can this happen to me?"; *"Who is to blame?"*

Once in the second stage, the individual recognizes that denial cannot continue. Because of anger, the person is very difficult to care for due to misplaced feelings of rage and envy. Any individual that symbolizes life or energy is subject to projected resentment and jealousy.

3. **Bargaining** —"Just let me live to see my children graduate."; "I'll do anything for a few more years."; "I will give my life savings if . . ."
   The third stage involves the hope that the individual can somehow postpone or delay death. Usually, the negotiation for an extended life is made with a higher power in exchange for a reformed lifestyle. Psychologically, the individual is saying, "I understand I will die, but if I could just have more time . . ."

4. **Depression** —"I'm so sad, why bother with anything?"; "I'm going to die . . . What's the point?"; "I miss my loved one, why go on?" During the fourth stage, the dying person begins to understand the certainty of death. Because of this, the individual may become silent, refuse visitors and spend much of the time crying and grieving. This process allows the dying person to disconnect oneself from things of love and affection. It is not recommended to attempt to cheer up an individual who is in this stage. It is an important time for grieving that must be processed.

5. **Acceptance** —"It's going to be okay."; "I can't fight it, I may as well prepare for it. "This final stage comes with peace and understanding of the death that is approaching. Generally, the person in the fifth stage will want to be left alone. Additionally, feelings and physical pain may be non-existent. This stage has also been described as the end of the dying struggle.

Kübler-Ross originally applied these stages to people suffering from terminal illness, later to any form of catastrophic personal loss (job, income, freedom). This may also include significant life events such as the death of a loved one, divorce, drug addiction, an infertility diagnosis, as well many tragedies and disasters.

Kübler-Ross claimed these steps do not necessarily come in the order noted above, nor are all steps experienced by all patients, though she stated a person will always experience at least two.

Often, people will experience several stages in a "roller coaster" effect—switching between two or more stages, returning to one or more several times before working through it.[2]

Significantly, people experiencing the stages should not force the process. The grief process is highly personal and should not be rushed, nor lengthened, on the basis of an individual's imposed time frame or opinion. One should merely be aware that the stages will be worked through and the ultimate stage of "Acceptance" will be reached.

However, there are individuals who struggle with death until the end. Some psychologists believe that the harder a person fights death, the more likely they are to stay in the denial stage. If this is the case, it is possible the ill person will have more difficulty dying in a dignified way. Other psychologists state that not confronting death until the end is adaptive for some people.[2] Those who experience problems working through the stages should consider professional grief counseling or support groups.

Cultural relevance

A dying individual's approach to death has been linked to the amount of meaning and purpose a person has found throughout their lifetime. A study of 160 people with less than three months to live showed that those who felt they understood their purpose in life, or found special meaning, faced less fear and despair in the final weeks of their lives than those who had not. In this and similar studies, spirituality helped dying individuals deal with the depression stage more aggressively than those who were not spiritual. [2]

NOTE: Author's Comment: A convenient way to remember Dr. Kubler Ross' Stages of Death and Dying would be to use the acronym DABDA, i.e.

D = Denial; A= Anger; B = Bargaining; D = Depression; A = Acceptance

This article uses bare URLs in its references. Please use proper citations containing each referenced work's title, author, date, and source, so that the article remains verifiable in the future. Help may be available. Several templates are available for formatting. (March 2010)

7. ^ "Milestones". TIME. Aug. 30, 2004. http://www.time. com/time/magazine/article/0,9171,689491,00.html.
8. ^ a b c d e Santrock, J.W. (2007). *A Topical Approach to Life-Span Development*. New York: McGraw-Hill. ISBN 0073382647.
9. ^ http://www.tc.columbia.edu/faculty/index. htm?facid=gab38 George A. Bonanno's Columbia University Faculty Page
10. ^ Bonanno, George (2009). *The Other Side of Sadness: What the New Science of Bereavement Tells Us About Life After a Loss*. Basic Books. ISBN 9780465013609. http://www.perseusbooksgroup.com/basic/book detail. jsp?isbn=0465013600.
11. ^ Maciejewski, P.K., *JAMA* (February 21, 2007). Retrieved April 14, 2009, http://jama.ama-assn.org/cgi/ content/abstract/297/7/716?etoc
12. ^ Friedman and James. "The Myth of the Stages of Dying, Death and Grief", *Skeptic Magazine* (2008). Retrieved 2008, from http://www.grief.net/Articles/Myth%20 of%20Stages.pdf

Further reading

• Kübler-Ross, E. (1973) *On Death and Dying*, Routledge, ISBN 0415040159

- Kübler-Ross, E. (2005) *On Grief and Grieving: Finding the Meaning of Grief Through the Five Stages of Loss*, Simon & Schuster Ltd, ISBN 0743263448
- Scire, P. (2007). "Applying Grief Stages to Organizational Change"
- *An Attributional Analysis of Kübler-Ross' Model of Dying*, Mark R Brent. Harvard University, 1981.
- *An Evaluation of the Relevance of the Kübler-Ross Model to the Post-injury Responses of Competitive Athletes*, Johannes Hendrikus Van der Poel, University of the Free State. Published by s.n., 2000.

External links

- Elisabeth Kübler-Ross Homepage
- Elisabeth Kübler-Ross—five stages of grief
- *On Death and Dying*—Interview With Elizabeth Kübler-Ross M.D.
  Beware the Five Stages of Grief—TLC Group Editorial

Retrieved from "http://en.wikipedia.org/wiki/K%C3%BCbler-Ross model"
Categories: 1969 books | Grief | Psychiatry works | Psychological theories | Psychology books | Self-help books

Interaction

- About Wikipedia
- Contact Wikipedia
- This page was last modified on 29 April 2010 at 13:44.
- Text is available under the Creative Commons Attribution-ShareAlike License; additional terms may apply. See Terms of Use for details.
- Wikipedia® is a registered trademark of the Wikimedia Foundation, Inc., a non-profit organization.

References

www.about.com

www.alllaw.com

www.bing.com/health

www.cms/gov/DualEligibility

www.fdhc.state.fl.us/
MedicaidMedicare.shtml

www.helpguide.org/Elder/

hospicecare.htm

www.hoke-eaeford.com

www.hospicefoundation.org

www.hospicepatients.org

www.longtermcarelink.net

www.medicaldictionary.com

www.retirementhomes.com

www.wiki.answers.com

www.abundanthealth4u.com

www.americanoutcomes.com

www.caringinfo.org

www.experc.mcw.edu

www.google.com

www.holisticmed.com

www.hospicefriends.net

www.hospicehomecares.org

www.hov.org

www.ll.en.wikipedia.org/wiki/
hospice

Free Encyclopedia

www.nywhatever.com

www.seniorcitizensguide.com

www.medicalterms.ws

Some Quotes used from:
When It's Time, Author, Dr. Curtis E. Smith, PUBLISHAMERICA
Publishing Company, 2008, Baltimore, MD, 197 pages, quoted from
pages 13-14, used with permission of author.

References

This article uses bare URLs in its references. Please use proper citations containing each referenced work's title, author, date, and source, so that the article remains verifiable in the future. Help may be available. Several templates are available for formatting. (March 2010)

13. ^ "Milestones". TIME. Aug. 30, 2004. http://www.time.com/time/magazine/article/0,9171,689491,00.html.
14. ^ *a b c d e* Santrock, J.W. (2007). *A Topical Approach to Life-Span Development.* New York: McGraw-Hill. ISBN 0073382647.
15. ^ http://www.tc.columbia.edu/faculty/index.htm?facid=gab38 George A. Bonanno's Columbia University Faculty Page
16. ^ Bonanno, George (2009). *The Other Side of Sadness: What the New Science of Bereavement Tells Us About Life After a Loss.* Basic Books. ISBN 9780465013609. http://www.perseusbooksgroup.com/basic/book_detail.jsp?isbn=0465013600.
17. ^ Maciejewski, P.K., *JAMA* (February 21, 2007). Retrieved April 14, 2009, http://jama.ama-assn.org/cgi/content/abstract/297/7/716?etoc
18. ^ Friedman and James. "The Myth of the Stages of Dying, Death and Grief", *Skeptic Magazine* (2008). Retrieved 2008, from http://www.grief.net/Articles/Myth%20of%20Stages.pdf

Further reading

- Kübler-Ross, E. (1973) *On Death and Dying,* Routledge, ISBN 0415040159
- Kübler-Ross, E. (2005) *On Grief and Grieving: Finding the Meaning of Grief Through the Five Stages of Loss,* Simon & Schuster Ltd, ISBN 0743263448

- Scire, P. (2007). "Applying Grief Stages to Organizational Change"
- *An Attributional Analysis of Kübler-Ross' Model of Dying*, Mark R Brent. Harvard University, 1981.
- *An Evaluation of the Relevance of the Kübler-Ross Model to the Post-injury Responses of Competitive Athletes*, Johannes Hendrikus Van der Poel, University of the Free State. Published by s.n., 2000.

External links

- Elisabeth Kübler-Ross Homepage
- Elisabeth Kübler-Ross—five stages of grief
- *On Death and Dying*—Interview With Elizabeth Kübler-Ross M.D.
Beware the Five Stages of Grief—TLC Group Editorial

References

Interaction

- About Wikipedia
- Contact Wikipedia
- This page was last modified on 29 April 2010 at 13:44.
- Text is available under the Creative Commons Attribution-ShareAlike License; additional terms may apply. See Terms of Use for details.
- Wikipedia® is a registered trademark of the Wikimedia Foundation, Inc., a non-profit organization.

From Wikipedia, the free encyclopedia

The **Health Insurance Portability and Accountability Act (HIPAA) of 1996 (P.L.104-191)** *[HIPAA]* was enacted by the U.S. Congress in 1996. It was originally sponsored by Sen. Edward Kennedy (D-Mass.) and Sen. Nancy Kassebaum (R-Kan.). According to the Centers for Medicare and Medicaid Services (CMS) website, Title I of HIPAA protects health insurance coverage for workers and their families when they change or lose their jobs. Title II of HIPAA, known as the Administrative Simplification (AS) provisions, requires the establishment of national standards for electronic health care transactions and national identifiers for providers, health insurance plans, and employers.

The Administration Simplification provisions also address the security and privacy of health data. The standards are meant to improve the efficiency and effectiveness of the nation's health care system by encouraging the widespread use of electronic data interchange in the U.S. health care system

What are the signs of approaching death?
In: Death and Dying [Edit categories]
Hospice & End Stage Help

152

Hospice and Caregiver Support Information on End of Life Stages
www.tlchomehospice.com/hospice.html

References

Licensed Vocational Nurse aka Licensed practical nurse

From Wikipedia, the free encyclopedia

Licensed Practical Nurses (LPNs) are also known as **Licensed Vocational Nurses (LVNs)** in California and Texas and as **registered practical nurses (RPNs)** in Ontario, Canada. They are called **enrolled nurses (ENs)** in Australia and New Zealand and as **state enrolled nurses (SENs)** in the United Kingdom.

United States

Main article: Nursing in the United States

Licensed Vocational Nurse (LVN) aka Licensed Practical Nurse (LPNs) works in a variety of health care settings, including Hospice Care. They are often found working under the supervision of physicians in clinics and hospitals, or in private home health care. In long term care facilities, they sometimes supervise nursing assistants and orderlies.

The United States Department of Labor's Bureau of Labor Statistics estimates that there are about 700,000 persons employed as licensed practical and licensed vocational nurses in the U.S.LVN and LPNs follow the rules of State Boards of Nursing. Requirements for taking boards usually include a clean criminal record and graduation from an approved accredited practical nursing program.

Education and training, depending on state requirements, may be vocational-based, hospital based, or college-based, and can vary from 9 month certificate programs to 3 years in time for certain specialties like pediatrics, surgery/anesthesia, or school nursing which usually require an associate degree in practical nursing.[1]

In Hospice Programs the LVN works directly under the supervision of a Registered Nurse (RN) sharing a patient case load. Generally, (with some exceptions) they perform the same Medical Services for patient care as the Registered Nurse (RN) Case Manager.

Resources

This article uses bare URLs in its references. Please use proper citations containing each referenced work's title, author, date, and source, so that the article remains verifiable in the future. Help may be available. Several templates are available for formatting. (March 2010)

19. ^ "Milestones". TIME. Aug. 30, 2004. http://www.time. com/time/magazine/article/0,9171,689491,00.html.
20. ^ *a b c d e* Santrock, J.W. (2007). *A Topical Approach to Life-Span Development*. New York: McGraw-Hill. ISBN 0073382647.
21. ^ http://www.tc.columbia.edu/faculty/index. htm?facid=gab38 George A. Bonanno's Columbia University Faculty Page
22. ^ Bonanno, George (2009). *The Other Side of Sadness: What the New Science of Bereavement Tells Us About Life After a Loss*. Basic Books. ISBN 9780465013609. http://www.perseusbooksgroup.com/basic/book_detail. jsp?isbn=0465013600.
23. ^ Maciejewski, P.K., *JAMA* (February 21, 2007). Retrieved April 14, 2009, http://jama.ama-assn.org/cgi/ content/abstract/297/7/716?etoc
24. ^ Friedman and James. "The Myth of the Stages of Dying, Death and Grief", *Skeptic Magazine* (2008). Retrieved 2008, from http://www.grief.net/Articles/Myth%20 of%20Stages.pdf

Further reading

- Kübler-Ross, E. (1973) *On Death and Dying*, Routledge, ISBN 0415040159
- Kübler-Ross, E. (2005) *On Grief and Grieving: Finding the Meaning of Grief Through the Five Stages of Loss*, Simon & Schuster Ltd, ISBN 0743263448

- Scire, P. (2007). "Applying Grief Stages to Organizational Change"
- *An Attributional Analysis of Kübler-Ross' Model of Dying*, Mark R Brent. Harvard University, 1981.
- *An Evaluation of the Relevance of the Kübler-Ross Model to the Post-injury Responses of Competitive Athletes*, Johannes Hendrikus Van der Poel, University of the Free State. Published by s.n., 2000.

External links

- Elisabeth Kübler-Ross Homepage
- Elisabeth Kübler-Ross—five stages of grief
- *On Death and Dying*—Interview With Elizabeth Kübler-Ross M.D.
Beware the Five Stages of Grief—TLC Group Editorial

Retrieved from "http://en.wikipedia.org/wiki/K%C3%BCbler-Ross model"
Categories: 1969 books | Grief | Psychiatry works | Psychological theories | Psychology books | Self-help books

Interaction

- About Wikipedia
- Contact Wikipedia
- This page was last modified on 29 April 2010 at 13:44.
- Text is available under the Creative Commons Attribution-ShareAlike License; additional terms may apply. See Terms of Use for details.
- Wikipedia® is a registered trademark of the Wikimedia Foundation, Inc., a non-profit organization.

Resources

1. NHPCO Facts & Figures, 2004. Alexandria, VA: National Hospice and Palliative Care Organization; 2004. Most current version is available at: http://www. nhpco.org/files/public/Statistics_Research/NHPCO_ facts-and-figures_2008.pdf. Accessed April 16, 2009.
2. Kinzbrunner BM, et al. 20 Common Problems in End-of-Life Care. New York, NY: Mc-Graw Hill; 2002.
3. Code of Federal Regulations, Title 42—Public Health. Chapter IV—Health Care Financing Administration, Department of Health and Human Services. Subchapter B—Medicare Program, Part 418—Hospice Care.

- Home (**Hospice Foundation of America**)

  Hospice Foundation of **America** is a not-for-profit organization that provides leadership in the development and application of **hospice** and its philosophy of care. Through programs . . . www.**hospicefoundation**.org · Cached page

  - Hospice Info
  - Order Products
  - DVDs
  - E-Newsletter
  - Grant Programs
  - Press Releases
  - The Dying Process
  - End Of Life

- Annual Educational Program (Education)

  Hospice Foundation of **America** is a not-for-profit organization that provides leadership in the development and application of **hospice** and its philosophy of care. Through and programs . . .

www.**hospicefoundation**.org/pages/page.asp?page_
id=65770 · <u>Cached page</u>

- **<u>Hospice Foundation</u> of America**

  Hospice Foundation of **America** online store—**Hospice Foundation** of **America** is a not-for-profit organization that provides leadership in the development and application of **hospice** . . .
  store.**hospicefoundation**.org · <u>Cached page</u>

- <u>American **Hospice Foundation**</u>

  American Hospice Foundation. Our Mission: To improve access to quality **hospice** care through public education, professional training, and advocacy on behalf of consumers.
  www.**americanhospice**.org · <u>Cached page</u>

- **<u>Hospice</u>** <u>Directory</u>

  In no way does a **hospice** represent an endorsement by the **Hospice Foundation** of **America**. **HFA** is a 501(c) (3) non-profit charitable organization and is not affiliated with any . . .
  www.**hospice**directory.org · <u>Cached page</u>

- **<u>Hospice Foundation</u> of America** : <u>Books</u>
  Hospice Foundation of **America** online store—**Hospice Foundation** of **America** is a not-for-profit organization that provides leadership in the development and application of **hospice** . . .
- store.**hospicefoundation**.org/home*<u>ahf@americanhospice. orgahf@americanhospice.org</u>*

- **<u>Hospice</u>** <u>Law,</u> **<u>Regulations</u>** <u>and federal laws</u>

More on this page

You can rest assured that the Federal and State governments have specific standards of care written into law to protect you and your loved one. Federally recognized **hospice** care in the United States began with implementation of parts of the Social Security Act (including Sections 1102, 1861 and 1871/42 U.S.C. 1302 and 1395hh and other sections).

Popular links

- State Websites
- Disclaimer
- Euthanasia Issues
- Find Attorney
- Find Hospice

Hospice law, **regulations** and federal laws govern the services that must be provided to **Hospice** patients, families and caregivers, set **Hospice** standards of care, describe **Hospice** . . .
www.**hospice**patients.org/hospic38.html ·Cached page

- **Hospice Regulations** and Notices

This list includes proposed and final **regulations** and notices about Medicare **Hospice** Payment.
www.cms.gov/**Hospice**/RegsNotices/list.asp · Cached page

- List of Websites for State **Hospice Regulations**

Listing of the website for each state's **hospice regulations**

APPENDAGE

<u>POLST?</u>   **For more information go to Website: Polst Task Force** www.polst.org

WHAT <u>IS</u> <u>POLST</u>?   **POLST**: An acronym for:

> **P**hysician
> **O**rder for
> **L**ife Sustaining
> **T**reatment

POLST History: In 1991 the **POLST** Philosophy was developed and began in the state of Oregon.

It was subsequently expanded to more than half of US states.

POLST: What is POLST?

- A Medical doctor's Order throughout the medical industry
- Portable documentation that transfers with the patient
- Completion of a POLST Form is Voluntary
- Allows individuals to choose medical treatment they want, and to identify those they do not want
- Provides specific directions to health care providers during serious illness

WHO Needs **POLST?**

- An individual with a terminal progressive illness
- An individual with a serious acute health condition
- A medically frail patient
- Criteria for Determining need: A life-limiting illness

POLST Requirements may vary from state to state

POLST Form Completion by Patient / Family is **VOLUNTARY**

POLST Does **NOT** Replace the Patient's **ADVANCE DIRECTORY**, it **COMPLEMENTS** it

A COPY of the **POLST Should** be kept in the **Patient's Medical Chart Record**

CONCLUSION

All information presented in this publication, A Hospice Guide Book; *Hospice Care, A Wise Choice,* is *not intended* as a substitute for information about Hospice Medical advice, and the reader should *not take any action* before consulting with a Hospice Professional and / or Medical doctors.

The purpose and goal of writing this book is to educate the public at large about Hospice, thus, enabling those who could become Hospice patients the opportunity to receive the benefit of expert comfort care, pain control management, symptom control, emotional, spiritual and psychosocial support, as they live with their terminal illness, during the end-of-life's journey, and peacefully transition from this life to the next.

At the risk of being redundant, it is again stated, the purpose for writing and publishing this book is to educate, enlighten, and inform the general public about Hospice care. It is not intended to be inclusive, nor does it attempt to give medical advice. Rather, the goal is to set down all in one place, cogent available information about Hospice care in a clear, concise, understandable way, thus, enabling the information to be *understood by all*.

If it satisfies that purpose, the effort, energy, and time spent researching and writing this book has been well rewarded, the purpose fulfilled, and the goal will have been met.

ABOUT THE AUTHOR

The Rev. Dr. Curtis E. Smith is a psychotherapist and an ordained, non-denominational Minister, who has worked with terminally ill hospice patients for the past twenty-three years.

His first book titled, *"When It's Time,"* is written about the counselor / patient relationship and specifically, patient attitude and thinking about their relationship to a Higher Power. Dr. Smith holds graduate degrees in marriage and family counseling, religious education, and human behavior. He also holds post-graduate degrees in psychology, religion and human behavior.

"Dr. Curtis," as he is fondly called by associates, colleagues, and patients, has extensive Education and experience in both acute hospital care and hospice settings, with Brea Community Hospital, Brea, California, where he served for eight years as resident Staff Chaplain, and with Cancer Treatment Centers of America, who was at that time, also occupied a wing located in Brea Community Hospital. He currently works with a national Health Care Hospice Agency organization, with offices in Southern California.

He is a published author and has written articles on death and dying, marriage, family, and religious articles dealing with life, spirituality and infinity. He has a Clinical Pastoral Educational background having trained with a Clinical Pastoral Education training Center with the Crystal Cathedral located in Garden Grove, California.

For twenty plus years, Dr. Curtis Smith was in private practice working as a Clinical Pastoral Psychotherapist with a Clinical Psychologist colleague, Dr. M. David Riggs, and Dr. Glenn Balch, Licensed Marriage, Family and Child Counselor. At one time they operated five Different offices located in Anaheim, Brea, Placentia, Yorba Linda, and Garden Grove, California.

This work about Hospice, titled: A Hospice Guide Book; *Hospice Care, A Wise Choice;* has been twenty years in the writing; this is Dr. Smith's second full length book.

Dr. Curtis Smith has worked for the past twenty-three in the Hospice Medical industry and is currently employed by one of the largest Healthcare Provider for both Home Care and Hospice Care in the United States. He resides with his family in Anaheim, California.

NOTES

Made in the USA
Lexington, KY
03 February 2012